This report contains the collective views of an international group of experts and does not necessarily represent the decisions or the stated policy of the World Health Organization

WHO Technical Report Series
899

CHEMISTRY AND SPECIFICATIONS OF PESTICIDES

Sixteenth report of the WHO Expert Committee on Vector Biology and Control

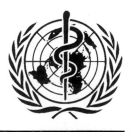

World Health Organization
Geneva 2001

WHO Library Cataloguing-in-Publication Data

WHO Expert Committee on Vector Biology and Control (1999 : Geneva, Switzerland)
    Chemistry and specifications of pesticides : sixteenth report of the WHO Expert
    Committee on Vector Biology and Control

(WHO technical report series ; 899)

1.Pesticides — chemistry 2.Pesticides — standards 3.Pest control — trends 4.Quality
control 5.Interinstituitional relations I.Title II.Series

ISBN 92 4 120899 6   (NLM classification : WA 240)
ISSN 0512-3054

The World Health Organization welcomes requests for permission to reproduce or translate its publications, in part or in full. Applications and enquiries should be addressed to the Office of Publications, World Health Organization, Geneva, Switzerland, which will be glad to provide the latest information on any changes made to the text, plans for new editions, and reprints and translations already available.

Typeset in Hong Kong
Printed in Singapore
2000/13239 — Best-set/SNP — 7000

Contents

WHO Expert Committee on Vector Biology and Control
Geneva, 6–10 December 1999

Members

Professor Atta-Ur-Rahman, Husein Ebrahim Jamal Research Institute of Chemistry, University of Karachi, Karachi, Pakistan

Dr M. Galoux, Department of Phytopharmacy, Ministry of Agriculture, Gembloux, Belgium (*Vice-Chairman*)

Dr D. Kanungo, Division of Agriculture and Cooperation, Directorate of Plant Protection, Quarantine and Storage, Central Insecticides Laboratory, Faridabad, India

Dr D.L. Mount, Centers for Disease Control and Prevention, Atlanta, GA, USA (*Rapporteur*)

Mr S.H. Tan, Pesticide Control Branch, Department of Agriculture, Jalan Gallagher, Kuala Lumpur, Malaysia (*Chairman*)

Representatives of other organizations

Food and Agriculture Organization of the United Nations (FAO)
Dr G. Vaagt, Pesticide Group, Plant Production and Protection Division, FAO, Rome, Italy

Global Crop Protection Federation
Dr T.S. Woods, Brussels, Belgium

Secretariat

Mr D.J. Hamilton, Animal and Plant Health Service, Department of Primary Industries, Brisbane, Australia (*Temporary Adviser*)

Dr A.R.C. Hill, Central Science Laboratory, Sand Hutton, York, England (*Temporary Adviser*)

Dr M. Zaim, Communicable Disease Control, Prevention and Eradication, WHO, Geneva, Switzerland (*Secretary*)

1. Introduction

The WHO Expert Committee on Vector Biology and Control met in Geneva from 6 to 10 December 1999. Dr Maria Neira, Director, Communicable Disease Control, Prevention and Eradication, opened the meeting on behalf of the Director-General. She noted that the Expert Committee had last considered the chemistry and specifications of pesticides in 1989 (*1*). Since then, there have been major changes in the approach, methods and means for vector and public health pest control. These include: further integration of vector control into basic health services; assumption of greater responsibility by individuals and communities for personal protection and vector control; improvement in pesticide formulation and application technology and, therefore, availability of safer, more acceptable and more effective pesticide products; and drastic changes in the pattern of use of pesticides by Member States for economic, human and environmental reasons.

Because of the increase in over-the-counter insecticide products for personal protection, greater attention must be given to human and environmental safety, packaging and labelling, and disposal of containers. It is also becoming increasingly important to harmonize, as far as possible, the specifications developed by WHO for public health pesticides with those of the Food and Agriculture Organization of the United Nations (FAO) for agricultural pesticides. WHO welcomes continued collaboration with FAO in that regard. However, specifications are developed for particular product uses, and careful attention has to be given to the different requirements of public health and agricultural pesticides.

The Expert Committee was therefore requested to:

— review trends in the use of pesticides (chemicals and formulations) for vector and public health pest control programmes and the development of quality control of pesticide products in the WHO Regions;
— review existing WHO specifications (full and interim) and test methods, and recommend changes; propose interim specifications that could be accepted as full specifications; and identify actions to be taken to upgrade the remaining interim specifications to full status;
— review the current status of specifications being developed for household insecticide products, bacterial larvicides and plant-based pesticides for public health use, and make recommenda-

tions on the establishment of WHO specifications for such products;

— review international rules/requirements for packaging, marking and storage of pesticides, and recommend actions to achieve the harmonization of international standards; and

— identify and discuss critical factors related to the disposal of unusable pesticides and pesticide containers.

The Expert Committee was requested to provide clear recommendations, in particular in regard to ways in which activities related to the WHO Pesticide Evaluation Scheme (WHOPES) and the technical support provided to Member States could be strengthened.

2. The WHO Pesticide Evaluation Scheme

The WHO Pesticide Evaluation Scheme (WHOPES), set up in 1960, is the only international programme that promotes and coordinates the testing and evaluation of pesticides intended for public health use. The International Code of Conduct on the Distribution and Use of Pesticides (2) constitutes the framework for WHOPES in promoting the safe handling and use, efficacy, cost–effective application and quality control of pesticide products/formulations for public health use. WHOPES develops specifications for pesticides and application equipment for use in international trade and quality control.

WHOPES functions in close collaboration with national disease and pest control programmes and national pesticide registration authorities, many international and regional organizations and institutions concerned with pesticide management, legislation and regulation, research institutions and with industry.

The global objectives of WHOPES are to:

— facilitate the search for alternative pesticides and application methodologies that are safe and cost-effective; and

— develop and promote policies, strategies and guidelines for the selective and judicious application of pesticides for public health use, and assist and monitor their implementation by Member States.

In its present form, established in 1982, WHOPES comprises a four-phase evaluation and testing programme.

Phase 1. Technical products or their formulations are tested for efficacy and persistence using laboratory-bred arthropods. This phase also comprises a study of cross-resistance with the various classes of pesticides currently available and the establishment of tentative diagnostic concentrations for the detection of vector resistance in the field. Compounds are also evaluated, in close collaboration with the International Programme on Chemical Safety (IPCS), for their safety for humans and the environment. Minimum laboratory experimentation to allow the confirmation of the basic toxicological and eco-toxicological information available from the manufacturer or other sources, in the light of the particular requirements of WHO, may also be carried out by appropriate WHO collaborating centres.

Phase 2. This phase comprises studies on natural vector populations in the field, on a small scale and under well-controlled conditions, to determine application doses and assess the efficacy and persistence of the product. Where appropriate, the action of products on non-target fauna is verified. Phase 2 is also the first opportunity to document any harmful effects of the product upon the operators in a field situation.

Phase 3. WHO, industry and one or more institutions located in disease endemic countries undertake to assess the efficacy of the product on a medium or large scale against a specified disease vector. Phase 3 comprises entomological, safety and, where appropriate, epidemiological evaluation. The institution supplies qualified staff for implementation, while the manufacturer supplies the insecticide and the funds needed for the trial. WHO bears the technical responsibility for the operation and is involved in the field through independent consultants. All three parties participate in drafting the trial protocol in accordance with a pre-established model that needs to be adapted to each situation. The final report is drafted by the institution, which submits it to WHO for evaluation. The report is then submitted for review to the manufacturer.

A scientific committee, the WHOPES Working Group, assists WHOPES in reviewing evaluation reports and assessing current knowledge about products for their intended applications, and makes recommendations to WHOPES on their public health use. The reports of the WHOPES Working Group meetings are issued as WHO documents and are widely distributed (*3–5*).

Phase 4. This phase is concerned with the establishment of specifications for the technical product and the formulations evaluated. Draft specifications proposed by industry are reviewed by members of the WHO Expert Advisory Panel on Vector Biology and Control and WHO collaborating centres and are then issued as interim specifications. These are reviewed every five to six years by the WHO Expert Committee on Vector Biology and Control, which may recommend their publication as full WHO specifications. WHO specifications for pesticides (interim and full) are available on the Internet at http://www.who.int/ctd/whopes.

In order to strengthen WHOPES activities, a global network, the Global Collaboration for Development of Pesticides for Public Health (GCDPP), was established in 1997. Participants include universities and research institutions, regional and international organizations, national and government-supported agencies, and pesticide and pesticide application equipment manufacturers. One of the main functions of GCDPP is to serve as an advisory group to WHOPES in matters relating to the development and safe and proper use of pesticides within the context of the International Code of Conduct on the Distribution and Use of Pesticides and WHO's global disease control strategies.

Since the Expert Committee last considered the chemistry and specifications of pesticides in 1989, 12 pesticide products have been fully evaluated for vector control, mainly for indoor residual spraying and insecticide treatment of mosquito nets for malaria vector control; WHO specifications have been published for these products.

WHOPES is currently evaluating seven insecticide products for indoor residual spraying and insecticide treatment of mosquito nets for malaria and/or Chagas vector control, two insect repellents, and two insect growth regulator mosquito larvicides, with ongoing trials in 14 countries.

Guideline specifications for household insecticide products — mosquito coils, vaporizing mats, liquid vaporizers and aerosols, were drafted at a WHO informal consultation, held in Geneva from 3 to 6 February 1998 (6). The draft guidelines have been distributed to ministries of health and national registration authorities for comments and suggestions.

WHOPES has also drafted guideline specifications for bacterial larvicides for public health use, i.e. *Bacillus thuringiensis israelensis* (*Bti*) and *B. sphaericus*. At an informal consultation held in Geneva from 28 to 30 April 1999 (7), the use of bacterial larvicides in public health and their registration requirements, including quality control and safety aspects, were reviewed. In addition, the requirements and objectives for inclusion in the specifications of bacterial larvicides were also reviewed and guideline specifications for the most common formulations of bacterial larvicides were drafted. The draft guidelines have been distributed to Member States and relevant institutions for comments and suggestions.

These activities have enabled WHOPES to plan for the expansion of the Scheme to include the testing and evaluation of a greater variety of pesticides. In recent years, WHOPES has also vigorously promoted the use of WHO specifications for public health pesticides in accordance with the International Code of Conduct on Distribution and Use of Pesticides. Examples of such efforts include the development and wide distribution of guidelines for the purchase of pesticides for public health use, provision of access to WHO specifications for pesticides and their test methods on the Internet, and an increase in the number of WHO collaborating centres for quality control of pesticides (currently three).

WHOPES has also established a database, which will be made available on the Internet through the WHO web site in the near future. The database contains the basic information that vector control professionals need to know for the day-to-day use of pesticides that have successfully completed evaluation under the Scheme, including type of application, recommended use, selected physical and chemical properties, basic toxicology, storage and handling, and reported cases of resistance (per species and country).

3. Trends in the use of pesticides for vector and public health pest control programmes in the WHO Regions

3.1 African Region

The African Region is the WHO Region with the highest burden of tropical diseases. It is estimated that 80–90% of total clinical malaria cases (300–500 million) and malaria-related deaths (1.5–2.7 million) occur in Africa and about 55 million people are at risk of human African trypanosomiasis. Plague remains a public health problem in several countries, with around 1000 cases and 100 deaths yearly, and several countries in Central and Eastern Africa experience a high prevalence of onchocerciasis. Schistosomiasis and relapsing fever also add to the burden of tropical diseases, although they are endemic in more limited areas.

Chemical control is the most widely practised method for vector and pest control in the Region. However, appropriate pesticide use is hampered, inter alia, by the: lack of capacity, coordinated mechanisms and funding for the registration, purchase, application and quality control of products; absence of effective systems for monitoring use; and lack of implementation of existing rules and regulations.

The major classes of pesticides in use in the Region are organochlorine and organophosphorus compounds, carbamates, pyrethroids and bacterial larvicides. Organophosphorus compounds are the most common, followed by pyrethroids. Insecticides are available in a variety of formulations, including emulsifiable concentrates (EC), wettable powders (WP), dustable powders (DP), suspension concentrates (SC), oil-in-water emulsions (EW) and capsule suspensions (CS).

Malaria vector control accounts for 80–90% of total pesticide use for public health purposes. Residual spraying uses the greatest volume of insecticides. However, the treatment of mosquito nets and other materials with pyrethroid insecticides is becoming an additional important method for personal protection and reduction of transmission of malaria.

DDT continues to be the pesticide most used in malaria vector control programmes in the Region with no significant decrease in overall quantities, although in some countries use has declined considerably. The introduction of insecticide-treated mosquito nets and the replacement of DDT by synthetic pyrethroids for indoor residual spraying have contributed to an increase in the public health use of pyrethroids.

In West Africa, the Onchocerciasis Control Programme is a major user of insecticides. More than 300000 litres of larvicides are applied each year. The use of organophosphorus compounds has progressively reduced, while that of bacterial larvicides has increased and now constitutes more than 50% of the total quantity of larvicides used in the Programme.

Plague control also requires large amounts of insecticides in certain countries. In Madagascar, 41825 kg of pyrethroid products were purchased for plague vector control in 1996 and an additional 5000 kg in 1997, while in Namibia, 18540 kg of insecticide products were used between 1993 and 1997.

Activities to control the vectors of schistosomiasis and human African trypanosomiasis remain limited but will be intensified in the future, particularly for tsetse fly control, for which insecticide-treated traps and screens represent the main method.

Pest control by municipalities and at household level accounts for a significant proportion of the overall use of pesticides.

Quality control of pesticides is an acute problem in Africa, particularly south of the Sahara. Few countries have established the functional mechanisms and structures required to undertake adequate quality control.

3.2 Region of the Americas

In many countries in Latin America vector-borne diseases such as malaria, dengue/dengue haemorrhagic fever, Chagas disease and leishmaniasis are still important causes of morbidity. In 1997, 1075445 cases of malaria and 741798 cases of dengue/dengue haemorrhagic fever were reported. In Brazil, 4% of the rural population are estimated to be positive for Chagas. Leishmaniasis, schistosomiasis and filariasis are important but localized problems. Control of these diseases relies on the integration of health and medical services with improved sanitation, house construction and the application of insecticides to reduce the contact of potential insect vectors with humans. Nevertheless, the use of pesticides remains a critical component in vector control programmes.

There has been a major shift in the quantities and types of pesticides used in vector control programmes, especially for malaria control. The number of houses sprayed each year for malaria control has decreased from a high of 15 million in 1964 to 1.6 million in 1997. The house spraying rate (number of houses sprayed per 1000 inhabitants) has also decreased from 100 in 1964 to 9 in 1997. The number of cases of malaria has increased from a low of 241462 in 1964 to just over one million cases in 1997.

The use of DDT for indoor residual house applications has been greatly reduced in the Region. In the 1970s, all of the 21 reporting countries were using DDT spraying as their primary control method against malaria. By 1997 only five countries, Argentina, Ecuador, Guyana, Mexico and Venezuela, reported the use of DDT. In the 1970s, organophosphorus, pyrethroid and carbamate insecticides were introduced by several countries as replacements for DDT. The combined total use of all of these is small compared to the quantities used when DDT was applied. This is due to a reduction in the number of houses treated and lower rates of application for the replacement insecticides.

Organophosphorus compounds such as malathion and fenitrothion were introduced in 1975 and remained in use in 1997 in seven countries. WP formulations are the most common for indoor residual applications. However, in some countries, notably Brazil and Mexico, malathion and fenitrothion ultra-low-volume (UL)[1] sprays and fogging have also been used as space sprays. In Brazil, malaria has been restricted to the Amazonian region, where precarious housing

---

[1] ULV has been commonly used as an abbreviation for ultra-low-volume formulations. The standard GCPF (formerly GIFAP) 2-character code is UL (8).

7

conditions provide few walls or surfaces that can be treated with insecticides. Space spraying, mainly in the form of thermal fogging, was introduced to reduce mosquito contact with the residents. In Manaus, north-west Brazil, malaria transmission also occurs in an urban setting. In several countries, especially in Central America, malaria control programmes have also included limited amounts of larviciding activities using temephos and fenthion.

WP formulations of carbamates such as propoxur and bendiocarb were previously used extensively for malaria control in Colombia, Costa Rica, El Salvador, Guatemala, Nicaragua and Panama, and sporadically in Mexico and Venezuela. The use of these products has been all but discontinued in the past 10 years except in Costa Rica and Guatemala, where they are still applied in small quantities.

Countries such as Costa Rica, El Salvador, Guatemala, Mexico, Nicaragua and Venezuela have used pyrethroids for indoor residual applications. Deltamethrin and λ-cyhalothrin have been the most commonly used. In Brazil, deltamethrin (SC and EC), cypermethrin (WP and SC), α-cypermethrin SC, λ-cyhalothrin WP and etofenprox WP have been used in different states for house applications. λ-Cyhalothrin EC, cypermethrin EC and deltamethrin fog EC have also been used in thermal fogging operations for malaria control.

Every country in Latin America and the Caribbean has at some time developed a national malaria control programme. In the past, these programmes were responsible for applying most of the insecticides used in public health. However, conventional indoor residual applications have now declined. Insecticide-treated mosquito nets have been used to a limited extent and several countries have used space spray applications as an alternative or supplement to residual applications. In southern Mexico, low-volume residual application of insecticides using motorized back-pack UL sprayers has been evaluated for malaria and dengue control.

The large programmes for control of Chagas disease in Argentina, Bolivia and Brazil use pyrethroids for indoor residual applications. Following the success of the campaign against the vector, *Triatoma infestans*, the number of houses treated in Brazil has been reduced.

Brazil is one of the few countries in the Americas that has applied insecticides for the control of visceral leishmaniasis (kala-azar). Since the areas of transmission often overlapped with those for Chagas disease, the insecticides used and areas sprayed were determined by the Chagas disease control programme. With the reduction in applications for Chagas disease control, the number of cases of kala-azar has increased and as a result many areas now require insecticide applications to reduce the incidence of this disease. Pyrethroids are applied at the rates established for Chagas control.

In the past 10 years, dengue has become increasingly important and large quantities of insecticides have been used to suppress country wide epidemics. Brazil has recently applied more insecticides for dengue control than for all of its other control programmes combined. The amounts of insecticide used for dengue control in other countries in the Region depend upon local conditions. Control of *Aedes aegypti*, the main vector, consists primarily of source reduction and focal treatment of breeding sites using temephos granules (GR). Thermal and UL space spraying are conducted in many countries on a routine and emergency basis. A variety of adulticides such as malathion, fenitrothion and deltamethrin have been used. These same insecticides have also been used in WP formulations for residual application to resting surfaces adjacent to larval breeding sites. The amount of insecticide used varies between countries, depending upon the levels of dengue and the importance given to its control. Brazil has the most extensive *A. aegypti* control programme in terms of coverage, budget, human resources and quantity of insecticide used.

3.3 Eastern Mediterranean Region

The most important vector-borne diseases in the Region are malaria, leishmaniasis, schistosomiasis, onchocerciasis, dengue, and other arboviral and rodent-borne diseases.

Malaria, transmitted by 18 anopheline mosquito species, continues to be a serious health problem in a number of countries, especially Afghanistan, Iraq, Somalia, Sudan and Yemen; an estimated 96% of Eastern Mediterranean malaria cases occur in these five countries. Overall an estimated 60% of the population of the Region are at risk of malaria.

Filariasis, transmitted mainly by culicine mosquitos, is limited to Egypt (Nile Delta), Somalia and Sudan. Both cutaneous and visceral leishmaniasis are present in the Region. The disease is of serious public health concern in six countries, Islamic Republic of Iran, Iraq, Saudi Arabia, Sudan, Syrian Arab Republic and Tunisia, and is present to a lesser degree in other countries.

Schistosomiasis is a serious health problem throughout much of the Region. Arboviral diseases such as dengue, Crimean-Congo haemorrhagic fever and Rift Valley fever are also found; dengue is an emerging disease in the Region. Plague remains a constant threat in some countries.

In principle, most countries have adopted integrated vector control as a strategy; however, in the absence of fully developed alternative vector and pest control methods, most continue to rely mainly on chemical pesticides.

The use of organochlorine insecticides, especially DDT, which is used against the vectors of malaria and leishmaniasis as an indoor residual spray, has been drastically reduced in recent years, with estimated applications for public health use of 168, 121 and 68 tonnes of active ingredient in 1989, 1992 and 1997, respectively. Most vector and pest species have developed resistance to DDT, which has been replaced by malathion and fenitrothion. The amounts of malathion used, mainly for the control of malaria vectors, are estimated to be 1814, 823 and 714 tonnes of active ingredient in 1989, 1992 and 1997, respectively. Development of resistance to malathion in the early 1980s in major anopheline mosquito vectors of malaria and the refusal of householders to accept indoor residual spraying because of the bad odour have resulted in a decline in the use of malathion. In general, there is a reduction in the use of organophosphorus insecticides in the Region; application of fenitrothion and pirimiphos-methyl is estimated to have fallen by 66% and 93%, respectively, between 1992 and 1997. This decrease appears to be mainly due to toxicity and higher costs for purchase and application.

There has been a significant upward trend in the use of various kinds and quantities of pyrethroids with a rise from an estimated 8.4 tonnes of active ingredients of all pyrethroids in 1992 to 22.3 tonnes in 1997.

Organophosphorus and pyrethroid insecticides are being used for indoor residual and space spraying for the control of malaria and other vectors and pests of public health importance.

The use of the larvicide temephos has been constantly on the increase in the Region, with estimated applications of 29, 300, 478 and 551 tonnes of active ingredient in 1979, 1989, 1992 and 1997, respectively.

So far, no serious resistance against pyrethroids has been recorded in vectors or pest populations, although there is an indication that it may be developing in some species. At present, 14 anopheline malaria vector species have developed resistance to organochlorine insecticides, eight to organophosphorus compounds and three to carbamates, and three species have reduced susceptibility to permethrin.

In recent years there has been a rapid increase in the use of insect growth regulators and bacterial larvicides.

Quality control of pesticides is generally weak in the Region but a number of national health authorities have requested technical support from the Regional Office for analysis of pesticides prior to bulk purchase. The Regional Office has designated the Regional Collaborating Centre in Pakistan as a focus for support for pesticide analysis and quality control.

3.4 South-East Asia Region

Vector-borne diseases continue to be a major public health problem in this Region. Approximately 1000 million people are living in malaria endemic areas and about 3 million malaria cases are reported annually to WHO; epidemics are common. Dengue/dengue haemorrhagic fever is the second most important vector-borne disease. During 1996–1998, most countries in the Region, with the exception of Bangladesh, Bhutan and Nepal, reported large outbreaks. It is estimated that 1330 million people are at risk in the Region. Lymphatic filariasis and Japanese encephalitis are endemic, and epidemics of the latter are common. Filariasis is endemic in eight Member States and current estimates suggest that up to 600 million people are at risk of infection. Approximately 50% of the global burden of lymphatic filariasis (60 million cases) presently occurs in this Region. Kala-azar has increased in the border areas between Bangladesh, India and Nepal, in part owing to the reduction in indoor residual spraying for malaria control.

Malaria control programmes are largely dependent on indoor residual spraying. Insecticide-treated mosquito nets and biological control using larvivorous fish have been promoted but are not used extensively at present. Response to dengue/dengue haemorrhagic fever epidemics depends largely upon space spraying while source reduction and larviciding, mainly using temephos and bacterial larvicides, have remained the methods of choice during inter-epidemic periods. Vector control measures against Japanese encephalitis likewise rely mainly on space spraying in affected areas. Although filariasis control depends mostly on case-finding and treatment, control of the major vector, *Culex quinquefasciatus*, through the application of larvicides and environmental management in urban areas has been practised. Control of kala-azar is fully dependent on indoor residual spraying of insecticides.

A wide range of insecticides from all major groups is used for public health purposes. For malaria control, only WP formulations are used for indoor residual spraying, while EC formulations are used as larvicides. UL and thermal fogging with malathion or pyrethroids have been used during malaria epidemics. For insecticide-treated mosquito net programmes, liquid (SC, EW and CS) formulations of pyrethroids are used.

Malaria control accounts for most of the insecticides used for public health purposes in the Region, which include DDT, organophosphorus and carbamate compounds and pyrethroids. In 1990, seven countries were still using DDT for malaria and/or kala-azar control. By 1997 only three countries, India, Myanmar and Thailand, continued to use DDT against malaria, while Bangladesh reserved DDT for kala-azar. Overall insecticide consumption during this period declined from 13319 to 7665 tonnes per year. Annual malathion consumption has declined sharply from 4157 tonnes of formulations to only 469 tonnes over the period 1981–1988. The total amount of fenthion used in India and Indonesia has increased from 4061 tonnes in 1990 to 7140 tonnes in 1997. In addition, fenitrothion was introduced to Indonesia in 1987 and Sri Lanka in 1994. Increasing attention is being given to the use of insecticide-treated mosquito nets, particularly in areas of moderate and low transmission. Only synthetic pyrethroids are being used and increasing consumption rates are anticipated.

Except for malaria, only limited information is available on the quantities of insecticides used for particular vector-borne disease control programmes and other public health purposes, but it has been observed that large amounts are being used for dengue vector control.

Biological larvicides have been introduced for malaria and dengue control in many countries. Locally manufactured biological larvicides are available. Personal protection measures have been promoted by control programmes, including the use of insect repellents, mosquito coils, mats and aerosols. Household pesticide use is increasing in India, Indonesia, Sri Lanka and Thailand.

3.5 Western Pacific Region

Malaria is the most important vector-borne disease in the 27 countries of the Region. The overall number of cases reported from the nine malaria endemic countries has been reduced by nearly 80% since 1992, but more than 400000 cases and 2000 deaths are still reported annually. Dengue/dengue haemorrhagic fever, the second most important vector-borne disease, occurs throughout the Region, resulting in significant morbidity and mortality. Schistosomiasis, lymphatic filariasis and various arboviral diseases also constitute problems in some countries.

For malaria control, insecticide-treated mosquito nets constitute the main control strategy. Coverage continues to increase, with some of the smaller countries approaching levels exceeding 85%. Of the estimated population at risk of 107 million, more than 23 million were protected by insecticide-treated mosquito nets by the end of 1998. Permethrin and deltamethrin in different formulations are the two insecticides used in most countries for mosquito net treatment.

As a consequence of the introduction of treated mosquito nets, the areas covered by residual spraying of houses have been greatly reduced. Only China, Malaysia, Solomon Islands and Viet Nam still have some regular indoor residual spraying programmes. DDT remains the primary insecticide for residual spraying but is being phased out in favour of the synthetic pyrethroids, mainly deltamethrin and λ-cyhalothrin. In 1997, Malaysia, which had undertaken regular indoor residual spraying with DDT for 26 years, switched to deltamethrin. In other countries, such as the Solomon Islands, the change from DDT to λ-cyhalothrin has been gradual. In some countries this has occurred as existing stocks of DDT have become depleted. Larviciding for anopheline mosquito control with temephos or *Bti* is generally limited.

For dengue, space spraying is used for epidemic control. Malathion, previously the insecticide of choice for dengue control, is slowly being replaced by pyrethroids, including a water-based formulation (EW). Larvicides including temephos and *Bti* are also used for the control of the two main vectors, *A. aegypti* and *A. albopictus*. Limited temephos resistance has been reported but does not appear to be a major problem.

The trend in insecticide use for malaria and dengue control is away from organochlorine and organophosphorus insecticides towards pyrethroids. The combined total of formulated organochlorine insecticide formulations used in the Region dropped from 162000kg in 1993 to 2000kg in 1998. Similarly, the total amount of formulated organophosphorus compounds applied dropped from 69000 to 18000kg during the same period. In contrast, the total amount of formulated pyrethroids used jumped from 56000 to 155000 litres. For malaria control, the shift towards pyrethroids is clearly due to the rapid switch from residual spraying to the use of insecticide-treated mosquito nets as the main form of vector control. The replacement of malathion by pyrethroids for space spraying for dengue control has also contributed to the trend. This is expected to continue as public health programmes shift towards more ecologically friendly formulations. However, the increased dependence on pyrethroids increases the risk of development of resistance to those compounds in vector populations.

Personal protection measures to prevent mosquito bites are actively used by householders. In many developed and medium-income countries in the Region, the use of household insecticide products constituted a major component of the total public health use of pesticides. The mosquito coil is used widely, followed by mats, aerosols and liquid vaporizers. The use of mosquito coils has increased every year from 1995 to 1997; China is the major user. Data indicate that the biggest market for household insecticide products is China, where in 1998 more than 10 000 million units of household insecticide products were used.

3.6 Common issues

The Committee identified the following common issues of importance related to the public health use of pesticides.

- Vector-borne diseases continue to be of global public health importance.

- There is continued reliance on chemical control of vectors.

- Current monitoring for insecticide resistance management of vectors and pests of public health importance is inadequate.

- Very few new cost–effective chemical pesticides suitable for public health use have been developed in recent years. Increasing reliance on pyrethroids raises concern with regard to the development of vector resistance to these compounds.

- Many countries are undergoing health sector reforms that pose new challenges in the selection, purchase, procurement, use and monitoring of insecticide application.

- The information currently available to WHO on the types and amounts of household, public health and agricultural pesticides used is limited. Such information is essential for proper pesticide management.

- Regulations for the control of pesticides exist in most countries, but enforcement of these regulations is frequently ineffective.

- Monitoring of the quality of pesticides used in public health programmes is limited.

- In some areas where there has been a reduction in the public health use of insecticides, there has been an increase in the incidence of vector-borne diseases. However, owing to the complexity of some situations, causal relationships have not always been established.

In light of these issues, the Committee recommended the following actions:

1. WHO should establish effective and sustainable vector resistance monitoring and reporting mechanisms, and develop guidelines on vector resistance management, with special emphasis on pyrethroids. The search for alternative, safe and cost–effective pesticides and control methods should receive high priority. This includes the search for alternatives to existing larvicides for addition to drinking-water for mosquito control.

2. The use of public health and agricultural pesticides should be monitored by WHO at the national level to assist in developing resistance management strategies and guidelines on the safe and proper use of pesticides, and agreements on pesticide usage at the international level.

3. WHO should conduct studies to determine whether there are causal relationships between changes in the patterns of chemical control of vectors and variations in the incidence of certain vector-borne diseases. For reasons of safety and economy, studies should be carried out to determine the cost-effectiveness of current vector control practices and to find ways of using pesticides more judiciously.

4. Countries should adopt a multisectoral approach to decision-making on pesticide management and strengthen their capacity to conduct appropriate vector control programmes at national and district levels. They should ensure that national pesticide regulations are enforced. Monitoring of the quality of pesticides used in public health programmes should be given high priority for reasons of safety and cost-effectiveness.

5. Public education on the safe and proper use of household pesticide products is of increasing importance. National authorities, international organizations and industry should play an active role in this area.

6. To maximize the useful lives of pesticides (i.e. the time before resistance reduces effectiveness) and to promote the cost–effective and safe use of available pesticide products, countries should establish national insecticide policies and guidelines on the use of pesticides in public health.

4. Analytical methods and quality control of pesticides in developing countries

Good product quality is essential to the effective and safe use of pesticides. Applying products that are lower in active ingredient content than declared could result in monetary loss and the application of a sublethal dose of pesticide, leading to ineffective control and promotion of the development of resistance. Products or formulations with inferior physicochemical properties such as suspensibility, emulsification or particle size characteristics, can also result in inadequate application and possibly increase the degree of risk for personnel, who may come into greater contact with the pesticide and/or pesticide-contaminated application equipment. Impurities formed during manufacture of the pesticide or by interaction in unstable formulations can increase product toxicity. Mislabelled or inadequately labelled products can cause various application and safety problems. In several surveys where pesticide samples were collected for testing from several sources in various countries around the world that lacked adequate quality control capacity, an average of one-third of the samples tested were found to be of substandard quality (9, 10). The proportion of substandard products collected from certain sources approached 90%. Reports on quality control testing, from countries where quality control capability has been established, indicate that the proportion of substandard products can be significantly reduced when adequate quality control is in place (B.-Y. Oh, 1999; A. Hourdakis & A. Alivizatos, 1999; A. Kouppari & A. Constantinou, 1999; T. Aye, 1999; and M. Chowdhury & W. Rahman, 1999, unpublished reports to WHOPES). Thus, there is an urgent need to make quality control capacity available to all countries currently lacking access to the necessary analytical facilities.

An effective quality control programme is expensive to establish and maintain; it involves the use of expensive reagents and equipment and requires operation by personnel with substantial training and expertise who can achieve credible, precise and accurate results. It is likely that the establishment of effective quality control capacity in many countries currently lacking such facilities will require assistance by outside groups with the necessary analytical expertise and possible financial support. For the past few years the Deutsche Gesellshaft für Technische Zusammenarbeit (GTZ) had assisted in the provision and establishment of quality control capacity in various countries, but has recently discontinued this support programme. One important aspect of this programme was the proficiency testing of pesticide quality control laboratories. There is an urgent need for this testing to continue and the Committee recommended that a strong effort be made to enlist the support of other international organizations to enable this programme to continue.

WHO regional collaborating centres for the quality control of pesticides have been established in Argentina, Belgium and Pakistan to provide the relevant facilities to countries with pesticide quality control needs in their regions. Such centres are needed to:

— validate results or serve in disputes
— maintain and distribute analytical standards throughout the region
— provide a clearing house for information
— test samples when requested by a country.

The Committee discussed the need to establish more regional collaborating centres to provide a better response to regional needs. However, concern was expressed that the current centres were underused, mainly because national policy-making, regulatory and purchasing authorities: were not aware of the possible prevalence of substandard products on the market, or the possible expense and problems associated with purchasing and using such products; were not aware of the quality control services provided by such centres; or expected a slower than needed or desired turn-around of the results.

The Committee concluded that efforts were needed to:

— raise the awareness of regulatory and purchasing authorities concerning pesticide quality control
— strengthen the current WHO collaborating centres with additional support
— try to find ways to reduce the expense and effort in collecting and shipping samples to the collaborating centres for testing
— assess, through WHO regional offices, the need for additional collaborating centres.

5. Specifications for pesticides

Testing of pesticide products is important because, where products meet their specifications, they can be expected to be effective and to pose no unexpected risks in use.

Where products do not comply with specifications, they should not be purchased and regulatory authorities should take appropriate action. Where products already held by the end-user fail to meet specifications, decisions on what to do with them can only be made on a case-by-case basis. End-users in this situation should take steps to avoid the problem in future by: purchasing products of good quality only; improving storage conditions; and/or using products within two years or before the expiry date (whichever is the sooner).

5.1 Synthetic pesticides

The Committee considered the harmonization of specifications issued by WHO and FAO. Many pesticides marketed internationally are of interest to both organizations, particularly insecticides and rodenticides. For some of these pesticides, WHO and FAO have published separate specifications, but the parameters to be measured and the criteria adopted are sometimes quite different. In most cases, it would be better to specify the same tests in both sets of specifications, particularly for technical materials (TC) and technical concentrates (TK). Because the intended functions of the formulated products may differ for agricultural and public health use, it is to be expected that the criteria (i.e. the limits quoted) for a particular type of formulation may also differ in some cases.

In 1999, FAO adopted a new procedure for establishing FAO specifications which was used for the specifications detailed in the most recent edition of its *Manual on the development and use of FAO specifications for plant protection products* (8). It requires more information to be provided by manufacturers ("minimum data package") before the adoption of a specification, and the specification developed applies only to the products submitted by the proposer(s). Subsequent proposers must prove the equivalence of their own products. The Committee considered that WHO should adopt the same process and that, as far as practicable, the development of specifications should be coordinated between the two Organizations. This would require the joint development of specifications for TC and TK.

With this approach, WHO and FAO specifications would have equal standing and equal transparency in development, and their acceptance would be enhanced. They could be used throughout the world with the same requirements concerning, for example, the tolerances on active ingredient content, impurities and the physicochemical tests required.

The Committee expressed concern at the fact that different chemical and physicochemical test methods are recommended by WHO and FAO. The FAO specifications give references to official and collaboratively tested methods adopted by the Collaborative International Pesticide Analytical Council (CIPAC) or by AOAC International (AOAC) and published by these organizations but do not provide full texts of the methods. In WHO specifications published up to 1997, the chemical and physicochemical methods are described in full, with the specifications, or under the heading "WHO test methods" in the same document. In some new Interim Specifications there are references to CIPAC methods, which are available only in the CIPAC Handbooks.

Harmonization of methods is important for the laboratories given the task of monitoring products for compliance with specifications, especially where they have to monitor pesticides for both public health and agricultural use. It would also enable the wider use of robust methods, validated by international collaborative studies.

After considering these general issues, the Committee made the following recommendations.

1. WHO and FAO should use a common system for the development of specifications and, as far as practical, all TC and TK specifications should be common to pesticides intended for both public health and agricultural use.

2. Specifications for formulated products of pesticides intended for both public health and agricultural use should include similar parameters, although the criteria may differ, according to the intended use.

3. Test methods intended for the support of WHO and FAO specifications should be common to both, where practicable. In this context, CIPAC and/or FAO should be asked to consider harmonization of the waters stipulated in their specifications with WHO standard waters.

4. WHO and FAO specifications made available on the Internet should be cross-referenced by means of hyperlinks, as appropriate.

5. WHO should adopt published CIPAC and AOAC International methods suitable for the support of specifications (see also recommendation 2 in section 8.3 of this report concerning the copyright of published methods).

6. Specifications should incorporate only the parameters to be tested and the corresponding quality criteria. Essential information on packaging, labelling, analytical and physical test methods should be included in annexes to the specifications.

7. WHO should draw to the attention of organizations such as CIPAC and AOAC International the fact that the quantities of analytical standards required to prepare calibration solutions are generally excessive in many published methods. The use of a more accurate balance and correspondingly smaller volumes of solvent for dilution will enable laboratories to prepare standards freshly and more economically.

8. The published list of common names and chemical names of pesticides contained in Annex 1 of *Specifications for pesticides used in public health: insecticides, molluscicides, repellerts, methods (11)* should be reformatted to make the presentation clearer. After the common name, the International Organization for Standardization (ISO), International Union of Pure and Applied Chemistry (IUPAC) and Chemical Abstract (CA) names should be printed with the Chemical Abstract Service (CAS) number and the CIPAC number.

5.2 Bacterial larvicides

The Committee considered the report of the WHO informal consultation on guideline specifications for bacterial larvicides for public health use, held in Geneva from 28 to 30 April 1999 (7), and reviewed the comments on the report and suggestions received from Member States and industry. The Committee made the following recommendations.

1. Industrial firms should be encouraged to develop test methods for accelerated storage stability determination for bacterial larvicides.

2. The industry should be encouraged to evaluate the applicability of CIPAC and WHO test methods for quality control of bacterial larvicides.

3. WHO and FAO should harmonize their efforts for development of specifications for biopesticides.

4. WHO regional collaborating centres should be designated to assist Member States in quality control of bacterial larvicides.

5. WHO/IPCS should develop guidelines in respect of maximum allowable microbial contaminants for bacterial larvicide products.

6. Industry should provide the relevant test methods to determine the identity and content of the active ingredients of bacterial larvicide products.

7. The biopotency limit requirements of $\pm 10\%$, specified in the report of the WHO informal consultation, may not be realistic; more collaborative testing is required to determine appropriate limits.

The Committee noted that the comments received indicated that the guidelines were timely and useful. However, the time available for the distribution of the consultation report and the receipt of comments from Member States had been limited. The Committee therefore recommended the further consideration of the report in future WHO consultations.

5.3 Plant-based pesticides

A number of plants have found use in different parts of the world for their pesticidal constituents. For example, *Azadirachta indica* Juss. (neem) preparations are marketed in the United States of America, Europe and Asia for use on both non-edible and edible crops. The growth in popularity of organic farming and organic food has further enhanced the importance of these materials.

The use of plant-based pesticides presents a number of challenges and advantages:

- The active ingredients of many plant-based pesticides are not known, but are essential for the development of specifications.

- The active ingredients can vary both in composition and concentration in the same plant species, in different clones, in different parts of the plants, at different stages of plant growth and under different climatic and soil conditions.

- The activity may not be due to a single ingredient but to a mixture of compounds, which may act synergistically.

- The development of resistance to pesticides containing a mixture of active ingredients may occur less readily.

- Adequate toxicological and ecotoxicological data are not available for many plant-based pesticides.

- Analytical standards of the active ingredients may not be easily obtainable.

Noting the above, the Committee made the following recommendations:

1. Collaborative testing procedures should be developed for plant-based pesticides. In this context it was noted that FAO is already processing a request for a specification for a plant-based pesticide.

2. WHO collaborating centres could be associated with the development of specifications of plant-based pesticides in collaboration with other organizations.

5.4 Household insecticide products

The increasing awareness and worsening situation of household pest problems and the improved socioeconomic conditions in many tropical developing countries have resulted in the increased demand and use of household insecticide products.

Although there are existing but limited national specifications for some of these products, there are no internationally agreed guideline specifications. A WHO informal consultation on guideline specifications for household insecticide products was held in Geneva from 3 to 6 February 1998, and draft guidelines (7) were circulated to Member States and industry for comments. The draft guidelines have generally met with overall approval and acceptance by national authorities and industry.

The Committee considered the draft guidelines and comments received by WHO and recommended that, with the following amendments, they should be accepted as the WHO guideline specifications for household insecticide products:

- For mosquito coils, the tolerance for the average weight of coil should be amended from ±1% to ±10% owing to the diverse materials used in manufacture, which vary from batch to batch.

- For mosquito coils and vaporizing mats, the term "mosquito repellent" should be included on the label.

- For aerosols, the storage stability test should be carried out at $40 \pm 2°C$ for 8 weeks or at $35 \pm 2°C$ for 12 weeks, where required.

- For aerosols, the maximum safe fill should be amended from 90% to 92.5% at 30°C.

The Committee agreed that the new harmonized flammability test under development by the United Nations Committee of Experts on the Transport of Dangerous Goods should be used when available. The Committee also noted that further collaborative work is required for the determination of droplet size for aerosol products. In addition, the Committee decided that differentiation between residual and space sprays should be maintained.

6. Containers, packaging, marking and storage of pesticides

The storage stability of a pesticide formulation depends on the intrinsic stability of the active ingredient, the formulation and the protective function of the packing material.

The pesticide container is essential in protecting the environment from the product, i.e. from leaks or spills caused by rough handling or pressure build-up in the container. The container must also protect the formulation from the environment, i.e. from moisture, or from air where the product is sensitive to oxygen. The container should not allow pressure on the product, which may result in caking.

Containers should not become brittle or corrode during prolonged storage. Pesticides should be expected to be fit for use after storage in unopened original containers for at least two years, unless labels state a shorter interval.

Where large quantities of pesticides are to be stored, a pesticide store should be designed to minimize potential accidents and environmental contamination.

Triple rinsing is generally effective in cleaning out and removing most of the pesticide from the container.

Pesticide containers must be labelled with information on the nature of the contents, instructions for the user, storage instructions, environmental precautions, and actions to take in the event of suspected poisoning.

Pesticides may be sold in packs of smaller packages for more convenience for the end-user. The smaller packages are referred to as packing units. The outer package should be designed so that the packing units remain intact and do not become contaminated on their surfaces.

The Committee recommended that industry ensure that containers for public health pesticides meet the following design characteristics and satisfy the needs of national registration and approval systems.

1. Pesticide containers must be sufficiently robust to protect the environment and people handling the containers from the product, i.e. from leaks, spills or rupture caused by rough handling or pressure build-up.

2. Containers must not contribute to formulation deterioration by allowing compression or moisture absorption during storage, which may result in caking or lumping.

3. Plastic containers must be designed to avoid brittleness and the tendency to crack during prolonged storage. The potential for brittleness is increased in a low-temperature environment.

4. The product/package combination must be designed for long-term storage under tropical and warm temperate conditions.

5. To ensure good rinsing characteristics, containers should be designed to comply with the United States Environmental Protection Agency (EPA) triple rinse test or other equivalent tests for their intended formulations, i.e. the fourth rinse with one-quarter of the container's volume is to contain no more than 0.0001% of the original concentration of active ingredient in the product.

The Committee recommended that product specifications stipulate those situations in which specific performance characteristics of the container are required (e.g. to avoid potential corrosion of metal containers or metal caps by the product during storage).

The Committee recommended that WHO provide training and education on the design of pesticide stores in order to minimize potential accidents and environmental contamination. Pesticide stores should be located away from residential areas and water courses; sites should be above flood height and cleared of vegetation and rubbish to reduce fire risk.

The Committee recommended that WHO prepare guidelines for the labelling of pesticides for public health use, which should be harmonized with the FAO guidelines on good labelling practice (*12*) while taking into consideration other international guidelines.

Pesticide labels should include sections on:

— product description and product category
— instructions for use
— user precautions
— instructions for storage
— date of release, manufacture or expiry date as applicable
— human and environmental safety precautions
— actions in the event of suspected poisonings, antidotes where applicable
— registration or approval number of the national authority
— emergency contact phone number of the manufacturer or designated representative in the event of spillage or fire.

Consideration should be given to the colour-coding of labels, and the use of pictograms and suitable language(s) on the label where culturally appropriate.

The Committee recommended that over-the-counter supply of pesticides for mosquito net treatment should include presentation in single-unit doses only, and that liquid formulations should be packaged in containers with child-proof caps.

The Committee discussed the value of expiry dates and their interpretation by users. An artificial disposal problem may arise if expiry dates are too conservative. Moreover, it is not clear whether the expiry date is set on the basis of expected diminished performance of the pesticide or on the basis of increased risk because of generation of toxic impurities. The Committee recommended that authorities setting expiry time intervals should evaluate the relevant data from industry and explain in a transparent way the basis for the expiry interval and the consequences for products that have passed their expiry date (lower potency, poor physical properties or generation of toxic impurities as an additional risk to users and bystanders).

7. Disposal of unusable pesticides and pesticide containers

Good practices in the management of pesticides include the avoidance or minimization of stocks of unusable pesticides.

The Committee noted the hazards associated with unusable pesticide stocks and the high cost of safe and environmentally sound disposal, and suggested that the long-term solution lies in preventive measures. The Committee recommended the following measures to avoid accumulation of unusable pesticides:

— provision of phasing-out when banning or deregistering pesticides
— investment in the building of proper and sufficient storage capacity
— training of staff in stock management, good storage practices and proper handling of pesticides during transport
— refusal of donations in excess of requirements
— the spelling out of product specifications, including required packaging and labelling (long-life labels), in tender documents or direct procurement orders.

Purchasers and users of public health pesticides should give high priority to such measures.

The problem of unusable pesticides, which are a source of environmental pollution as well as a threat to human health, is widespread and common and disposal of bulk quantities is sometimes necessary. The situation is most serious in developing countries where there is little awareness of the inherent dangers of pesticides, and the resources and expertise for handling such problems are very limited.

There are no easy disposal methods that are safe, economical and generally applicable under circumstances prevailing in developing countries. Conventional methods such as burning or burying of unused pesticides are not environmentally friendly because the end result may be damage to human health and the environment.

In the public health sector, the major users and custodians of pesticides are governments and governmental organizations. There are many reasons for accumulation of unusable pesticides, including the lack of harmonization between procurement and actual need. The general public are minor accumulators and custodians of unusable stocks of household pesticides. In this case the problem is less acute as the purchases are mostly related to small quantities and are needs based. The Committee suggested that regulation of the use, sale and stewardship of pesticide products should be extended to disposal of pesticides and pesticide containers.

With regard to available disposal options, a distinction must be made between small and large quantities of product to be disposed of. Certain disposal methods may be considered acceptable for small quantities, but not for large quantities. The health and environmental hazards connected to the product must also be taken into consideration.

There are several disposal methods that may be acceptable for specific types of products under certain local conditions. These include high-temperature incineration, chemical treatment and specially engineered landfill. There are also several promising new developments (e.g. gas-phase chemical reduction and plasma energy pyrolysis). However, it is essential to select the disposal method on a case-by-case basis.

The Committee made the following recommendations.

1. Prior to the registration of any new pesticide, the manufacturer should indicate a practical method of disposal.

2. WHO should encourage research into the development of cost–effective methods for disposal of bulk quantities of unusable and unwanted public health pesticides.

3. Old stocks of bulk pesticides should be analysed and tested wherever practical to determine whether they are still usable for their intended purpose.

4. Householders should be encouraged to use household pesticides for their intended purposes and to dispose of containers safely.

5. Clear instructions for container disposal should be given on the label.

6. All pesticide containers should be triple rinsed (preferably immediately after emptying) before disposal.

7. Empty pesticide containers should not be used for other purposes but should be returned to the manufacturer for recycling and disposal.

8. Collaboration with other organizations

8.1 Food and Agriculture Organization of the United Nations

The Committee expressed its appreciation for the continuing intensive collaboration between FAO and WHO and endorsed the envisaged further expansion of this cooperation to reflect the guiding role of these two organizations in the implementation of the International Code of Conduct on the Distribution and Use of Pesticides.

The Committee made the following recommendations.

1. The specification guidelines described in Chapters 4–6 of the FAO publication *Manual on the development and use of FAO specifications for plant protection products* (8) should be adopted for pesticides used both in public health and agriculture, those used exclusively in agriculture and those used exclusively in public health.

2. FAO and WHO (WHOPES) should use the same definitions, nomenclatures, format and supporting methodologies for pesticide specifications.

3. FAO and WHO (WHOPES) should develop joint specifications for technical materials (TC) and technical concentrates (TK) for those pesticides used in both public health and agriculture.

4. Joint projects should be established between FAO and WHO (WHOPES) to strengthen the capacity of national and subregional analytical laboratories for pesticide quality control. In addition, both organizations should explore the possibility of other joint projects to support the implementation of the Code of Conduct.

8.2 Global Crop Protection Federation

The Global Crop Protection Federation (GCPF) (formerly the International Group of National Associations of Manufacturers of Agrochemical Products, GIFAP), which represents national associations of pesticide producers, informed the Committee of its appreciation for the invitation by WHO to participate in the process of setting WHO specifications for products for use in public health programmes, and expressed its willingness, in principle, to cooperate with WHO to ensure that the process is effective and efficient. GCPF is especially encouraged by the stated intent of WHO to harmonize its specifications process with that of FAO. Such harmonization is desirable to minimize duplication of effort and to gain maximum benefit from resources dedicated to the specification-setting process. Moreover, GCPF is also willing, in principle, to participate in efforts required to solve other technical problems identified by WHOPES, and which are deemed relevant by GCPF members.

The Committee recommended that, in cooperation with industry, FAO and WHO (WHOPES and IPCS) should develop procedures for joint evaluation of data and publication of specifications for technical and formulated pesticides.

8.3 Collaborative International Pesticides Analytical Council and AOAC International

There has been long-term and fruitful collaboration between WHOPES, CIPAC and AOAC International in support of analytical methods for quality control of WHO specifications.

CIPAC confirmed its continuing collaboration with WHO and particularly with the WHOPES programme.

The Committee made the following recommendations.

1. The relationships between WHOPES and CIPAC and AOAC International should be strengthened and formalized to promote the optimum use of resources in preparing and using analytical and test methods.

2. Agreements should be developed between WHOPES and CIPAC and AOAC International for the reprinting/publication of CIPAC and AOAC International methods in WHO pesticide specifications.

8.4 International Union of Pure and Applied Chemistry

The IUPAC Commission on Agrochemicals and the Environment seeks to advance research understanding and promote environmental stewardship and human safety with agrochemicals through its publications, international pesticide congresses and regional workshops. The Committee was informed that IUPAC has taken the decision to become a project-driven body and is seeking relevant project proposals from outside organizations such as WHO and FAO.

Commission projects currently in progress include studies on: the relevance of impurities in technical-grade pesticides; the disposal and degradation of pesticide waste; and regulatory limits for pesticide residues in water.

The Committee recommended that WHOPES should consider proposing projects to or seeking expert advice from IUPAC on issues relevant to pesticides used in public health.

9. General recommendations

In concluding its work, the Committee made the following general recommendations.

1. To improve further the quality of pesticides used in public health, WHO should ensure the wide distribution of WHO specifications and should strengthen and expand pesticide quality control programmes. For reasons of human and environmental safety, efficacy and economy, pesticide products of good quality are essential.

2. Where pesticides must be used in public health, WHO, in collaboration with industry and other relevant institutions, should further promote safety and judicious use.

3. To ensure harmonization of procedures used in the development of specifications for agricultural and public health pesticides, collaborative efforts between WHO and FAO should be further strengthened and formalized. Such harmonized procedures will: improve the quality of the specifications; enhance their acceptability by governments, industry and traders; provide transparency to the process and the decisions; and make the development of such specifications more efficient and cost-effective to industry and to FAO and WHO.

4. WHO should facilitate and promote the search for alternative pesticides and control measures that pose minimal risk to human health and the environment, and are cost-effective. In this context, further strengthening of collaboration with relevant research institutions and industry should be sought.

5. Considering the limited number of pesticides developed in recent years and the need to extend the useful life of the available compounds, WHO, in collaboration with other relevant institutions, should strengthen pesticide resistance monitoring in vectors and pests of public health importance and promote effective and practical resistance management strategies.

6. To improve the management of pesticides globally, WHO and FAO, with the assistance of industry and national authorities, should promote intersectoral programmes for monitoring the use of agricultural, public health and household pesticides.

Acknowledgements

The Expert Committee acknowledges the valuable contributions of the following WHO staff members, which helped to provide a basis for its discussions and report: Dr A.T. Aitio, International Programme on Chemical Safety, World Health Organization, Geneva, Switzerland; Dr C. Frederickson, Regional Adviser, WHO Regional Office for the Americas/PAHO, Brasília, Brazil; Dr P. Guillet, Communicable Disease Control, Prevention and Eradication, World Health Organization, Geneva, Switzerland; Dr L. Manga, Regional Adviser, WHO Regional Office for Africa, Harare, Zimbabwe; Dr M. Nathan, Communicable Disease Control, Prevention and Eradication, World Health Organization, Geneva, Switzerland; Dr K. Palmer, Regional Adviser, WHO Regional Office for the Western Pacific, Manila, Philippines; Dr C. Prasittisuk, Regional Adviser, WHO Regional Office for Souith-East Asia, New Delhi, India; Dr H. Rathor, Regional Adviser, WHO Regional Office for the Eastern Mediterranean, Alexandria, Egypt.

References

1. *Chemistry and specifications of pesticides. Thirteenth report of the WHO Expert Committee on Vector Biology and Control.* Geneva, World Health Organization, 1990 (WHO Technical Report Series, No. 798).

2. *International Code of Conduct in the Distribution and Use of Pesticides.* Rome, Food and Agriculture Organization of the United Nations, 1990.

3. *Report of the first WHOPES Working Group meeting: WHO/HQ, Geneva, 26–27 June 1997.* Geneva, World Health Organization, 1997 (unpublished document CTD/WHOPES/97.5; available on request from Communicable Disease Control, Prevention and Eradication, World Health Organization, 1211 Geneva 27, Switzerland).

4. *Report of the second WHOPES Working Group meeting: WHO/HQ, Geneva, 22–23 June 1998: review of alpha-cypermethrin 10% SC and 5% WP cyfluthrin 5% EW and 10% WP.* Geneva, World Health Organization, 1998 (unpublished document CTD/WHOPES/98.10; available on request from Communicable Disease Control, Prevention and Eradication, World Health Organization, 1211 Geneva 27, Switzerland).

5. *Report of the third WHOPES Working Group meeting: WHO/HQ, Geneva, 23–24 September 1999: review of deltamethrin 1% SC and 25% WT etofenprox 10% EC and 10% EW.* Geneva, World Health Organization (unpublished document WHO/CDS/CPE/WHOPES/99.4; available on request from Communicable Disease Control, Prevention and Eradication, World Health Organization, 1211 Geneva 27, Switzerland).

6. *Draft guideline specifications for bacterial larvicides for public health use: report of the WHO informal consultation, 28–30 April 1999, WHO, Geneva.* Geneva, World Health Organization, 1999 (unpublished document WHO/CDS/CPC/WHOPES/99.2; available on request from Communicable Disease Control, Prevention and Eradication, World Health Organization, 1211 Geneva 27, Switzerland).

7. *Draft guideline specifications for household insecticide products: report of the WHO informal consultation 3–6 February 1998, WHO, Geneva.* Geneva, World Health Organization, 1998 (unpublished document CTD/WHOPES/IC/98.3; available on request from Communicable Disease Control, Prevention and Eradication, World Health Organization, 1211 Geneva 27, Switzerland).

8. *Manual on the development and use of FAO specifications for plant protection products*, 5th ed. Rome, Food and Agriculture Organization of the United Nations, 1999 (FAO Plant Production and Protection Paper, No. 149).

9. **Kern M, Vaagt G.** Pesticide quality in developing countries. *Pesticide Outlook*, 1996, *1*:1–10.

10. **von Dueszeln J, Vereno I, Wieland T.** Pesticide quality control — experiences from GTZ plant protection projects. *Agriculture and Rural Development*, 1995, **2**:37–40.

11. *Specifications for pesticides used in public health: insecticides, molluscicides, repellents, methods*, 7th ed. Geneva, World Health Organization, 1997, Annex 1 (unpublished document WHO/CTD/WHOPES/ 97.1; available on request from Communicable Disease Control, Prevention and Eradication, World Health Organization, 1211 Geneva 27, Switzerland).

12. *Guidelines on good labelling practice for pesticides.* Rome, Food and Agriculture Organization of the United Nations, 1995.

Annex 1
Recommended changes to existing specifications and methods

1. General changes to specifications

The Committee recommended the following changes in, or additions to, certain sections of the existing WHO specifications (*1–3*).

1.1 "Material" and "Description and ingredients"

The titles should be changed to "Description" and the relevant descriptions for different pesticide products given in the FAO *Manual on the development and use of FAO specifications for plant protection products (4)*.

1.2 Active ingredient content

The identity tests, range of declared contents and stated tolerances given in section 3.3 of the FAO Manual (*4*) should be adopted.

Declared content in g/kg or g/l at 20 °C ± 2 °C	Tolerance
Up to 25	± 15% of the declared content for homogeneous formulations or ± 25% for heterogeneous formulations
Above 25 up to 100	± 10% of the declared content
Above 100 up to 250	± 6% of the declared content
Above 250 up to 500	± 5% of the declared content
Above 500	± 25 g/kg or g/l

In each range the upper limit is included.

1.3 Impurities

The impurities included in a specification must be relevant and their inclusion justified. The maximum permitted level should normally be quoted as a percentage of the determined active ingredient content.

1.4 Physical and physicochemical properties

CIPAC test methods (*5*) should be referenced when available. If not, WHO test methods should be used and published.

1.4.1 *Temperature*

A temperature of 30 °C ± 2 °C should normally be used.

1.4.2 *Density*

A temperature of 20 °C ± 2 °C should normally be used.

1.4.3 *Suspensibility*

The words: "the tube must be isolated from hand's heat" should be deleted. Suspensibility should be tested after heat stability treatment. In case of unacceptable results, the suspensibility should be determined without heat treatment.

1.4.4 *Dustability*

The requirement for this test should be deleted. Consideration should be given to introducing the dry sieve test, as used for FAO specifications for dustable powder (DP) formulations (*4*).

1.4.5 *Water*

It is suggested that the standard soft water should contain 34.2 mg/kg calculated as calcium carbonate (WHO standard water), not 20.0 mg/kg (CIPAC standard water) and that the preparation of WHO standard hard water and WHO standard soft water should be published as WHO test methods (see Annex 2 in this report).

1.4.6 *Stability tests*

The requirements and wording of the FAO Manual (*4*) should be adopted.

Stability at $0\,°C \pm 2\,°C$ for 7 days: CIPAC method MT 39.3 (*5*)

Stability at elevated temperature: CIPAC method MT46 (*5*):
$54\,°C \pm 2\,°C$ for 14 days
$45\,°C \pm 2\,°C$ for 6 weeks
$40\,°C \pm 2\,°C$ for 8 weeks
$35\,°C \pm 2\,°C$ for 12 weeks
$30\,°C \pm 2\,°C$ for 18 weeks.

1.4.7 *Persistent foam*

WHO specifications for pesticides intended for dispersion/dilution in water should incorporate a specification for persistent foam, to minimize the potential for heterogeneous distribution of active ingredient and for contamination of the clothes and the skin of the user. CIPAC method MT 47.2 (*5*) and the method given in the FAO Manual (*4*) (maximum 60 ml after 1 minute) should be used.

1.4.8 *Wettability*

WHO specifications for dry products intended for dispersion in water (e.g. wettable powders and water-dispersible granules) should incorporate a specification for wettability, to ensure rapid wetting. CIPAC method MT 53.3 (*5*) and the method given in the FAO Manual (*4*) (normally the formulation shall be wetted in 1 minute without swirling) should be used.

1.4.9 *Flash-point*

Flash-point should be specified to the nearest degree Celsius.

1.4.10 *Sieving*

The sieve tests (wet and dry) should be conducted after heat stability treatment according to CIPAC methods MT 59, MT 167 and MT 170 (5). In case of unacceptable results, sieving should be determined without heat treatment.

1.4.11 *Methods*

Methods, requirements and descriptions should be harmonized in their format and content. For example:

- Description of the reagents or apparatus: replace "special reagents or apparatus" with "reagents or apparatus".

- It is not necessary to specify the minimum purity of calibration standards, although the purity must be known and the absence of interferences must be checked.

- Chromatographic columns: "or equivalent" should be specified, unless no alternative can be used.

- Presentation of injection sequences should be harmonized: calibration, sample, sample, calibration, ...

- Presentation of calculations and the expression of formulae principles should be harmonized.

1.4.12 *Analytical standards*

Laboratories should be reminded that, in case of difficulty in obtaining standards, industry and WHO collaborating centres may be able to provide these materials.

1.4.13 *Reference*

WHO specifications should provide cross-references to relevant information in IPCS and FAO documents and/or publications.

2. Specific changes to specifications

The Committee further recommended the following specific changes in, or additions to, certain specifications (*1–3*) in accordance with the general changes to specifications given in Annex 1, section 1.

The changes proposed should be circulated by WHO to industry for comment before final adoption.

2.1 Bendiocarb

Technical (TC)
    Content: see Annex 1, section 1.2.
    Melting-point: a melting range should be specified.

Water-dispersible powder (WP)
    Content: see Annex 1, section 1.2.
    Persistent foam: see Annex 1, section 1.4.7.
    Wettability: see Annex 1, section 1.4.8.
    Heat stability: see Annex 1, section 1.4.6.

Dustable powder (DP)
    Content: see Annex 1, section 1.2.
    Dustability: see Annex 1, section 1.4.4.
    Heat stability: see Annex 1, section 1.4.6.

Ultra-low-volume liquid (UL)
    Content: see Annex 1, section 1.2.
    Cold test: see Annex 1, section 1.4.6.
    Flash-point: see Annex 1, section 1.4.9.
    Heat stability: see Annex 1, section 1.4.6.

2.2 Brodifacoum

Technical (TC) — interim specification published in 1997 (2)
    Content: see Annex 1, section 1.2.

Accepted as full specification, subject to the amendment proposed.

Concentrates at 5g/kg and 25g/kg (TK) — interim specification published in 1997 (2)

Accepted as full specification.

Baits at 10mg/kg and 50mg/kg (RB) — interim specification published in 1997 (2)

Recommended for retention as interim specification because there is no accepted guideline for the specification of baits. Industry should be asked to propose a guideline specification for consideration by WHO and FAO.

2.3 Chlorpyrifos

Technical (TC)
    Content: see Annex 1, section 1.2.

Emulsifiable concentrate (EC)
    Content: see Annex 1, section 1.2.
    Cold test: see Annex 1, section 1.4.6.
    Flash-point: see Annex 1, section 1.4.9.
    Persistent foam: see Annex 1, section 1.4.7.
    Heat stability: see Annex 1, section 1.4.6.

2.4 Cyfluthrin

Technical (TC) — interim specification published in 1998 (*3*)
    Content: see Annex 1, section 1.2.

Accepted as full specification, subject to the amendment proposed.

Water-dispersible powder (WP) — interim specification published in 1998 (*3*)
    Wettability: see Annex 1, section 1.4.8.
    Sieving: Sieve mesh sizes should conform with FAO requirements (75 μm).
    Suspensibility: see Annex 1, section 1.4.3.

Recommended as interim specification, subject to resolution of sieve mesh size and incorporation of the amendments proposed.

Emulsion, oil in water (EW) — interim specification published in 1998 (*3*)

Accepted as full specification.

2.5 λ-Cyhalothrin

Technical (TC) — interim specification published in 1997 (*2*)
    Content: see Annex 1, section 1.2.

Accepted as full specification, subject to the amendment proposed.

Water-dispersible powder (WP) — interim specification published in 1997 (*2*)
    Persistent foam: see Annex 1, section 1.4.7.
    Wettability: see Annex 1, section 1.4.8.
    Sieving: see Annex 1, section 1.4.10.
    Suspensibility: see Annex 1, section 1.4.3.
    Heat stability: see Annex 1, section 1.4.6.

Accepted as full specification, subject to the amendments proposed.

Emulsifiable concentrate (EC) — interim specification published in 1997 (*2*)
    Content: see Annex 1, section 1.2.
    Persistent foam: see Annex 1, section 1.4.7.
    Cold test: see Annex 1, section 1.4.6.
    Heat stability: see Annex 1, section 1.4.6.

Accepted as full specification, subject to the amendments proposed.

2.6 α-Cypermethrin

Technical (TC) — interim specification published in 1998 (*3*)
    Content: see Annex 1, section 1.2.

Accepted as full specification, subject to the amendment proposed.

Water-dispersible powder (WP) — interim specification published in 1998 (*3*)
    Sieving: see Annex 1, section 1.4.10.
    Suspensibility: see Annex 1, section 1.4.3.

Accepted as full specification, subject to the amendments proposed.

Aqueous-suspension concentrate (SC) — interim specification published in 1998 (*3*)
    Suspensibility: see Annex 1, section 1.4.3.

Accepted as full specification, subject to the amendment proposed.

2.7 DDT

Refer to published capillary gas chromatography methods.

Water-dispersible powder (WP)
    p,p'-DDT content: see Annex 1, section 1.2.
    Persistent foam: see Annex 1, section 1.4.7.
    Wettability: see Annex 1, section 1.4.8.
    Suspensibility: see Annex 1, section 1.4.3.
    Heat stability: see Annex 1, section 1.4.6.

Water-dispersible powder (WP) for overseas shipment
    Delete specification since it is superfluous.

Emulsifiable concentrate (EC)
    Delete specification. DDT EC is not recommended by WHO for any purpose.

Dustable powder (DP)
    Content: see Annex 1, section 1.2.
    Sieving: see Annex 1, section 1.4.10.
    Dustability: see Annex 1, section 1.4.4.
    Heat stability: see Annex 1, section 1.4.6.

2.8 Deet

Technical (TC)
    Density: see Annex 1, section 1.4.2.

2.9 Deltamethrin

Technical (TC)
    Content: see Annex 1, section 1.2.

Water-dispersible powder (WP)
    Persistent foam: see Annex 1, section 1.4.7.
    Sieving: see Annex 1, section 1.4.10.
    Suspensibility: see Annex 1, section 1.4.3.
    Heat stability: see Annex 1, section 1.4.6.

Emulsifiable concentrate (EC)
    Content: see Annex 1, section 1.2.
    Cold test: see Annex 1, section 1.4.6.
    Heat stability: see Annex 1, section 1.4.6.

Dustable powder (DP)
    Content: see Annex 1, section 1.2.
    Sieving: see Annex 1, section 1.4.10.
    Dustability: see Annex 1, section 1.4.4.
    Heat stability: see Annex 1, section 1.4.6.

Ultra-low-volume liquid (UL)
    Content: see Annex 1, section 1.2.
    Cold test: see Annex 1, section 1.4.6.
    Flash-point: see Annex 1, section 1.4.9.
    Heat stability: see Annex 1, section 1.4.6.

Aqueous suspension concentrate (SC) — interim specification published in 1998 (3)
    Persistent foam: see Annex 1, section 1.4.7.

Accepted as full specification, subject to the amendment proposed.

2.10 Diazinon

CIPAC and manufacturers should be asked to modify the analytical method to use an alternative internal standard (aldrin specified). Methods are not available for impurities.

Water-dispersible powder (WP)
    Content: see Annex 1, section 1.2.
    Impurities: limits for O,S-TEPP and S,S-TEPP content should be set relative to the active ingredient content.
    Persistent foam: see Annex 1, section 1.4.7.
    Wettability: see Annex 1, section 1.4.8.
    Suspensibility: see Annex 1, section 1.4.3.
    Heat stability: see Annex 1, section 1.4.6.
    pH: wording should be changed to "not lower than 7 and not higher than 10.5".

Emulsifiable concentrate (EC)
    Content: see Annex 1, section 1.2.
    Persistent foam: see Annex 1, section 1.4.7.
    Cold test: see Annex 1, section 1.4.6.
    Heat stability: see Annex 1, section 1.4.6.

2.11 Dichlorvos

WHO should review the specifications to take account of the chloral impurity specification.

Technical (TC)
    Content: see Annex 1, section 1.2.

Emulsifiable concentrate (EC)
    Content: see Annex 1, section 1.2.
    Persistent foam: see Annex 1, section 1.4.7.
    Cold test: see Annex 1, section 1.4.6.
    Heat stability: see Annex 1, section 1.4.6.

2.12 Diflubenzuron

Technical (TC or TK)
    Note: owing to the presence of a stabilizer the specification relates
        only to the technical concentrate (TK).

    Content: see Annex 1, section 1.2.

Water-dispersible powder (WP)
    Content: see Annex 1, section 1.2.
    Persistent foam: see Annex 1, section 1.4.7.
    Sieving: see Annex 1, section 1.4.10.
    Suspensibility: see Annex 1, section 1.4.3.
    Heat stability: see Annex 1, section 1.4.6.

2.13 Dimethoate

The specification should be reviewed by WHO to take account of the iso-dimethoate and omethoate content.

Technical (TC)
    Content: see Annex 1, section 1.2.
    Method for impurity(ies): give reference to CIPAC method 59/TC/
        (M2) (6).

Emulsifiable concentrate (EC)
    Content: see Annex 1, section 1.2.
    Persistent foam: see Annex 1, section 1.4.7.
    Cold test: see Annex 1, section 1.4.6.
    Heat stability: see Annex 1, section 1.4.6.

2.14 Endosulfan

Technical (TC)
Content: see Annex 1, section 1.2.
Melting-point: a melting range should be specified.

Emulsifiable concentrate (EC)
Content: see Annex 1, section 1.2.
Persistent foam: see Annex 1, section 1.4.7.
Cold test: see Annex 1, section 1.4.6.
Heat stability: see Annex 1, section 1.4.6.

2.15 Etofenprox

Technical (TC) — interim specification published in 1997 (2)
Content: see Annex 1, section 1.2.

Accepted as full specification, subject to the amendment proposed.

Water-dispersible powder (WP) — interim specification published in 1997 (2)
Sieving: see Annex 1, section 1.4.10.
Suspensibility: see Annex 1, section 1.4.3.

Accepted as full specification, subject to the amendments proposed.

2.16 Fenitrothion

Technical (TC)
Content: see Annex 1, section 1.2.

Emulsifiable concentrate (EC)
Content: see Annex 1, section 1.2.
Persistent foam: see Annex 1, section 1.4.7.
Cold test: see Annex 1, section 1.4.6.
Heat stability: see Annex 1, section 1.4.6.

Water-dispersible powder (WP)
Content: see Annex 1, section 1.2.
Persistent foam: see Annex 1, section 1.4.7.
Sieving: see Annex 1, section 1.4.10.
Suspensibility: see Annex 1, section 1.4.3.
Heat stability: see Annex 1, section 1.4.6.

2.17 Fenthion

Technical (TC)
Content: see Annex 1, section 1.2.

Water-dispersible powder (WP)
    Content: see Annex 1, section 1.2.
    Persistent foam: see Annex 1, section 1.4.7.
    Wettability: see Annex 1, section 1.4.8.
    Sieving: see Annex 1, section 1.4.10.
    Suspensibility: see Annex 1, section 1.4.3.
    Heat stability: see Annex 1, section 1.4.6.

Emulsifiable concentrate (EC)
    Content: see Annex 1, section 1.2.
    Persistent foam: see Annex 1, section 1.4.7.
    Cold test: see Annex 1, section 1.4.6.
    Heat stability: see Annex 1, section 1.4.6.

2.18 Iodofenphos

Technical (TC)
    Content: see Annex 1, section 1.2.

Water-dispersible powder (WP)
    Content: see Annex 1, section 1.2.
    Persistent foam: see Annex 1, section 1.4.7.
    Wettability: see Annex 1, section 1.4.8.
    Sieving: see Annex 1, section 1.4.10.
    Suspensibility: see Annex 1, section 1.4.3.
    Heat stability: see Annex 1, section 1.4.6.

2.19 Lindane

Technical (TC)
    Content: see Annex 1, section 1.2.

Water-dispersible powder (WP)
    Content: see Annex 1, section 1.2.
    Persistent foam: see Annex 1, section 1.4.7.
    Wettability: see Annex 1, section 1.4.8.
    Sieving: see Annex 1, section 1.4.10.
    Suspensibility: see Annex 1, section 1.4.3.
    Heat stability: see Annex 1, section 1.4.6.
    Method: include reference to CIPAC method 488/TC/M3 (7).

Emulsifiable concentrate (EC)
    Content: see Annex 1, section 1.2.
    Persistent foam: see Annex 1, section 1.4.7.
    Cold test: see Annex 1, section 1.4.6.
    Heat stability: see Annex 1, section 1.4.6.
    Method: include reference to CIPAC method 488/TC/M3 (7).

Dustable powder (DP)
    Content: see Annex 1, section 1.2.
    Sieving: see Annex 1, section 1.4.10.
    Dustability: see Annex 1, section 1.4.4.
    Heat stability: see Annex 1, section 1.4.6.
    Method: include reference to CIPAC method 488/TC/M3 (7).

2.20 Malathion

WHO should review the specifications to consider clauses for iso-malathion for the TC, EC and DP.

Technical (TC)
    Content: see Annex 1, section 1.2.

Water-dispersible powder (WP)
    Content: see Annex 1, section 1.2.
    Persistent foam: see Annex 1, section 1.4.7.
    Wettability: see Annex 1, section 1.4.8.
    Sieving: see Annex 1, section 1.4.10.
    Suspensibility: see Annex 1, section 1.4.3.
    Heat stability: see Annex 1, section 1.4.6.

Emulsifiable concentrate (EC)
    Content: see Annex 1, section 1.2.
    Persistent foam: see Annex 1, section 1.4.7.
    Cold test: see Annex 1, section 1.4.6.
    Heat stability: see Annex 1, section 1.4.6.

Dustable powder (DP)
    Content: see Annex 1, section 1.2.
    Sieving: see Annex 1, section 1.4.10.
    Dustability: see Annex 1, section 1.4.4.
    Heat stability: see Annex 1, section 1.4.6.

2.21 Methoxychlor

Technical (TC)
    Content: see Annex 1, section 1.2.

Emulsifiable concentrate (EC)
    Content: see Annex 1, section 1.2.
    Persistent foam: see Annex 1, section 1.4.7.
    Cold test: see Annex 1, section 1.4.6.
    Heat stability: see Annex 1, section 1.4.6.

2.22 Niclosamide

WHO should review the specification to take account of the new CIPAC analytical method for niclosamide (ref. 4113/M, in press).

Technical ethanolamine salt (TC)
   Melting-point: A melting range should be specified.

   The calculation should be checked for the expression of niclosamide (not salt).

Water-dispersible powder (WP)
   Persistent foam: see Annex 1, section 1.4.7.
   Wettability: see Annex 1, section 1.4.8.
   Sieving: see Annex 1, section 1.4.10.
   Suspensibility: see Annex 1, section 1.4.3.
   Heat stability: see Annex 1, section 1.4.6.

Emulsifiable concentrate (EC)
   Content: see Annex 1, section 1.2.
   Persistent foam: see Annex 1, section 1.4.7.
   Cold test: see Annex 1, section 1.4.6.
   Heat stability: see Annex 1, section 1.4.6.

2.23 Permethrin

Technical (TC)
   Content: see Annex 1, section 1.2; the *cis*-isomer must be in the range 25–40% of the total permethrin isomer content.

Emulsifiable concentrate (EC)
   Content: see Annex 1, section 1.2.
   Persistent foam: see Annex 1, section 1.4.7.
   Cold test: see Annex 1, section 1.4.6.
   Heat stability: see Annex 1, section 1.4.6.

2.24 Phoxim

Technical (TC)
   Content: see Annex 1, section 1.2.

Emulsifiable concentrate (EC)
   Content: see Annex 1, section 1.2.
   Persistent foam: see Annex 1, section 1.4.7.
   Cold test: see Annex 1, section 1.4.6.
   Heat stability: see Annex 1, section 1.4.6.

2.25 Pirimiphos-methyl

Technical (TC)
   Content: see Annex 1, section 1.2.

Water-dispersible powder (WP)
    Content: see Annex 1, section 1.2.
    Persistent foam: see Annex 1, section 1.4.7.
    Wettability: see Annex 1, section 1.4.8.
    Sieving: see Annex 1, section 1.4.10.
    Suspensibility: see Annex 1, section 1.4.3.
    Heat stability: see Annex 1, section 1.4.6.

Emulsifiable concentrate (EC)
    Content: see Annex 1, section 1.2.
    Persistent foam: see Annex 1, section 1.4.7.
    Cold test: see Annex 1, section 1.4.6.
    Heat stability: see Annex 1, section 1.4.6.

2.26 Propoxur

Technical (TC)
    Content: see Annex 1, section 1.2.

Water-dispersible powder (WP)
    Content: see Annex 1, section 1.2.
    Persistent foam: see Annex 1, section 1.4.7.
    Wettability: see Annex 1, section 1.4.8.
    Sieving: see Annex 1, section 1.4.10.
    Suspensibility: see Annex 1, section 1.4.3.
    Heat stability: see Annex 1, section 1.4.6.

2.27 Pyrethrum

Technical concentrate (TK)
    Content: see Annex 1, section 1.2.

2.28 Temephos

Technical (TC)
    Content: see Annex 1, section 1.2.

Emulsifiable concentrate (EC)
    Content: see Annex 1, section 1.2.
    Persistent foam: see Annex 1, section 1.4.7.
    Cold test: see Annex 1, section 1.4.6.
    Heat stability: see Annex 1, section 1.4.6.

Emulsifiable concentrate for Simulium control (EC)
    Content: see Annex 1, section 1.2.
    Density: see Annex 1, section 1.4.2.

Sand granules (GR)
   Content: see Annex 1, section 1.2, except that the tolerance for a declared content of up to 25 g/kg should be ±25% owing to the heterogeneity of the product.

2.29 Trichlorfon

Technical (TC)
   Content: see Annex 1, section 1.2.

Water-soluble powder (SP)
   Content: see Annex 1, section 1.2.
   Sieving: see Annex 1, section 1.4.10.
   Heat stability: see Annex 1, section 1.4.6.

3. Specific changes to WHO test methods

The Committee made the following recommendations in relation to WHO test methods (*1*)

Sampling procedures (WHO/M/1)
The text of Note 1, page 103, of the FAO Manual (*4*) (sampling of SC) should be incorporated:

> Before sampling to verify the formulation quality, inspect the commercial container carefully. On standing, suspension concentrates usually develop a concentration gradient from the top to the bottom of the container. This may even result in the appearance of a clear liquid on the top and/or of sediment on the bottom. Therefore, before sampling, homogenize the formulation according to the instructions given by the manufacturer or, in the absence of such instructions, by gentle shaking of the commercial container (for example by inverting the closed container several times). Large containers must be opened and stirred adequately. After this procedure, the container should not contain a sticky layer of non-dispersed matter at the bottom. A suitable and simple method of checking for a non-dispersed sticky layer "cake" is by probing with a glass rod or similar device adapted to the size and shape of the container. All the physical and chemical tests must be carried out on a laboratory sample taken after the recommended homogenization procedure.

Visual suspensibility test for DDT WP 750 g/kg (WHO/M/2.R2)
The text of this method should be incorporated in the DDT specification. The method should be deleted.

Determination of acidity and alkalinity (WHO/M/3)
The method should be deleted. Reference to it should be replaced by reference to CIPAC method MT 31 (*5*).

Sieving test after heat stability treatment (WHO/M/4.R1)
The method should be deleted. Reference to it should be replaced by reference to CIPAC method MT 59 (*5*).

Determination of melting-point and mixed melting-point (WHO/M/5.R1)

The method should be deleted. Reference to it should be replaced by reference to CIPAC method MT 2 (5).

Karl Fischer electrometric titration method for determination of water content (WHO/M/7.R1)

The method should be retained and reference should also be made to the new CIPAC method MT 30.5 adopted in 1999 but not yet published.

Dean and Stark distillation method for determination of water content (WHO/M/8.R1)

The method should be deleted. Reference to it should be replaced by reference to CIPAC method MT 30.2 (5).

Determination of material insoluble in dichloro-difluoromethane (WHO/M/9)

The method should be deleted.

Tag-closed tester for determination of flash-point (WHO/M/10.R1)

The method should be deleted. Reference to it should be replaced by reference to CIPAC method MT 12 (5).

Cleveland open tester method for determination of flash-point (WHO/M/11.R1)

The method should be deleted.

Emulsion stability test (WHO/M/13.R3)

The method should be retained but CIPAC should be requested to harmonize the requirement for soft water with WHO. Re-emulsification at 24 hours should be required by WHO specifications.

Toxicity test for larvicidal oils (WHO/M/18)

The text of this method should be incorporated in the specifications. The method should be deleted.

Preparation and conditioning of gas–liquid chromatographic columns (WHO/M/20)

The method should be deleted.

Determination of material insoluble in acetone (WHO/M/21.R1)

The method should be deleted. Reference to it should be replaced by reference to CIPAC method MT 27 (5).

Viscosity (WHO/M/22)

The method should be deleted. Reference to it should be replaced by reference to CIPAC method MT 22 (5) for kinematic viscosity.

Cold test (WHO/M/23)
The method should be deleted. Reference to it should be replaced by reference to CIPAC method MT 39 (5).

Volatility (WHO/M/24)
The method should be retained.

pH (WHO/M/25)
The method should be deleted. Reference to it should be replaced by reference to CIPAC method MT 75 (5).

Hardness of water (WHO/M/26)
The method should be deleted. Reference to it should be replaced by reference to CIPAC method MT 73 (5).

4. New WHO test methods

The Committee recommended the following new methods (see Annex 2).

- Method for the determination of tablet disintegration time (not collaboratively tested).

- Method for the determination of tablet integrity (not collaboratively tested).

- Preparation of WHO standard hard water.

- Preparation of WHO standard soft water.

References

1. *Specifications for pesticides used in public health: insecticides, molluscicides, repellents, methods*, 7th ed. Geneva, World Health Organization, 1997 (unpublished document WHO/CTD/WHOPES/97.1; available on request from Communicable Disease Control, Prevention and Eradication, World Health Organization, 1211 Geneva 27, Switzerland).

2. *Interim specifications for pesticides used in public health.* Geneva, World Health Organization, 1997 (unpublished document WHO/CTD/WHOPES/97.7; available on request from Communicable Disease Control, Prevention and Eradication, World Health Organization, 1211 Geneva 27, Switzerland).

3. *Interim specifications for pesticides used in public health.* Geneva, World Health Organization, 1997 (unpublished document WHO/CTD/WHOPES/97.7; available on request from the Department of Communicable Disease Control, Prevention and Eradication, World Health Organization, 1211 Geneva 27, Switzerland).

4. *Manual of the development and use of FAO specifications for plant protection products*, 5th ed. Rome, Food and Agriculture Organization of the United Nations, 1999 (FAO Plant Production and Protection Paper, No. 149).

5. **Dobrat W, Martijn A.** *Physico-chemical methods for technical and formulated pesticides. CIPAC Handbook, Vol. F.* Cambridge, Black Bear Press, 1995.

6. **Dobrat W, Martijn A.** *Analysis of technical and formulated pesticides. CIPAC Handbook, Vol. H.* Cambridge, Black Bear Press, 1998.

7. **Dobrat W, Martijn A.** *Analysis of technical and formulated pesticides. CIPAC Handbook, Vol. 1G.* Cambridge, Black Bear Press, 1998.

Annex 2
Recommended specifications for new pesticides and formulations, and new methods

I. New pesticides and formulations

Deltamethrin water-dispersible tablets (WT)

Interim specification.[1]

1. Specification

1.1 Description

The material shall consist of a homogeneous mixture of technical deltamethrin together with carriers and any other suitable formulants. It shall be in the form of tablets or pills that disintegrate, disperse and wet out readily on stirring into water. The technical deltamethrin used in the manufacture of the water-dispersible tablets shall comply with the requirements of specification WHO/SIT/24.R1 (1).

1.2 Chemical and physical requirements

The material, sampled from any part of the consignment (see WHO method WHO/M/1 (1); see Annex 1, section 3, of this report), shall comply with the requirements of section 1.1 and with the following requirements.

---

[1] Retained as an interim specification pending collaboratively tested methods for disintegration time and tablet integrity.

1.2.1 *Deltamethrin content (g/kg basis)*

The content of deltamethrin, determined by the method described in section 2.1, shall not differ from the nominal content by more than the following amount:

Nominal content	Tolerance permitted
Up to 25 g/kg	±15% of the declared content
Above 25 g/kg up to 100 g/kg	±10% of the declared content
Above 100 g/kg up to 250 g/kg	±6% of the declared content

The average content of all samples taken shall not be lower than the nominal content.

1.2.2 *Deltamethrin R-isomer content (g/kg basis)*

The deltamethrin *R*-isomer content, determined by the method described in section 2.2, shall not be higher than 2% of the deltamethrin content found under section 1.2.1.

1.2.3 *Water content*

The water content, determined by CIPAC method MT 30 (*2*), shall not be higher than 20 g/kg.

1.2.4 *pH of aqueous dispersion*

The pH of an aqueous dispersion, determined by CIPAC method MT 75 (*2*), shall lie within the range of 4.0 to 6.0.

1.2.5 *Disintegration time*

The time taken to obtain a complete disintegration of the tablet when tested by WHO method WHO/M/28 (see Annex 2, section II) should not exceed 2 minutes 30 seconds.

1.2.6 *Wet sieve test*

Not less than 98% of the water-dispersible tablet shall pass through a 75-μm sieve after disintegration in water when tested by CIPAC method MT 59.3 (*2*).

1.2.7 *Tablet integrity*

No broken tablets shall be found when tested by WHO method WHO/M/27 (see Annex 2, section II). The degree of attrition shall be 2% maximum.

1.2.8 *Suspensibility*

When tested by the method described in section 2.3 equivalent to CIPAC method MT 15 (*2*), a minimum of 70% of the deltamethrin (0.035 g/l) shall be in suspension 30 minutes after agitation of a suspension containing deltamethrin at a concentration of 0.05 g/l prepared in WHO standard hard water (see WHO method WHO/M/29; see Annex 2, section II) at 30°C ± 2°C from the water-dispersible tablet.

Alternatively, if the buyer requires other standard waters or temperatures to be used, this shall be specified when ordering.

1.2.9 *Heat stability*

The water-dispersible tablet, after treatment as described in CIPAC method MT 46.1 (*2*), shall comply with the requirements of sections 1.2.1–1.2.5, 1.2.7 and 1.2.8 of this specification.

1.3 *Packing and marking of packages*

Each deltamethrin water-dispersible tablet shall be individually sealed in foil before placement in an outer pack.

Two pack sizes shall be available:

Loose tablets. Several foil-sealed tablets are packed loose in an outer cardboard pack. Full instructions for use and precautions are provided on the label on the outside of the pack and on several fly sheets (as specified in the order) packed inside the cardboard box with the tablets.

Envelope and presentation tablets. Single foil-sealed tablets are attached to an envelope card labelled with full instructions for use and precautions. Several envelope cards are packed in a single outer carton labelled with full instructions for use and precautions.

All packages shall bear, durably and legibly marked on the product label, the following:

— manufacturer's name
— "Deltamethrin water-dispersible tablet"
— "Deltamethrin. . . . g/kg"
— batch or reference number, and date of test
— net weight of contents
— date of manufacture
— instructions for use

and the following minimum cautionary notice:

Deltamethrin is a pyrethroid that acts predominantly on the central nervous system; high dosages have been found to cause toxic seizures in experimental animals. A high concentration in air may be irritant, and contact with the concentrated product may induce a temporary tingling sensation, particularly on the face. Deltamethrin may be hazardous if swallowed. Avoid skin contact; wear protective gloves and clean protective clothing when handling the product or dipping nets. Wash splashes from skin or eyes immediately with plenty of water. Wash hands and exposed skin thoroughly before meals and after use. Allow treated nets to dry and air thoroughly before use.

Keep packs out of the reach of children and well away from foodstuffs and animal feed and their containers.

Deltamethrin is hazardous to aquatic wildlife. Avoid accidental contamination of ponds, waterways or ditches with product or diluted material.

If poisoning occurs, call a physician. Treatment is symptomatic.

2. Methods of determining chemical and physical properties

2.1 *Deltamethrin content*

2.1.1 *Outline of method*

Note: The method used to determine the deltamethrin content differs slightly from the method described in the current WHO specification for deltamethrin technical and deltamethrin formulations (WP, EC, DP, UL, SC) in order to accommodate the extraction of deltamethrin active ingredient from the water-dispersible tablet.

Deltamethrin is extracted from the water-dispersible tablet sample with a mixture of dioxane and water. The suspension is further diluted five times with iso-octane and filtered. The deltamethrin content is determined by comparing the response of the sample with that of a deltamethrin standard by high-performance liquid chromatography (HPLC), using a Nucleosil column (or equivalent) and a mixture of dioxane and iso-octane as the mobile phase.

2.1.2 *Apparatus*

Liquid chromatograph. The instrument should be one that is designed for use with stainless steel columns and is equipped with: a pumping system able to maintain a pressure of 15 MPa; a UV spectrophotometer detector able to measure UV absorbance at 254 nm; and a loop-type injector.

Liquid chromatographic column. The column should be a stainless steel tube 20 cm long and 4.0 mm in internal diameter packed with Nucleosil 5 CN, 5 μm, Macherey Nagel (720007) or equivalent.

Recorder. 1-mV full-scale sensitivity, or integrator.

2.1.3 *Reagents*

Deltamethrin standard. Analytical grade, of known purity.

1,4-Dioxane. HPLC grade. Check the peroxide content and purity if necessary. Dioxane is mixed with water at a concentration of 1.5 ml/l before use.

Iso-octane. HPLC grade.

Mobile phase. A degassed mixture of 6 ml of dioxane and 94 ml of iso-octane. Diluting solvent: dioxane–iso-octane 20:80 (v/v).

2.1.4 *Preparation of the calibration solution*

Weigh (to the nearest 0.1 mg), in duplicate, about 50 mg of delta-methrin standard into two 50-ml volumetric flasks (C_1 and C_2). Add to both flasks a small amount of diluting solvent (20 ml of dioxane + 80 ml of iso-octane) and shake the flasks to dissolve the standard. Dilute to volume with the same solvent and mix thoroughly.

2.1.5 *Operating conditions for high-performance liquid chromatography*

The conditions given below are typical values and may have to be adapted to obtain optimal results from a given apparatus.

Column temperature (oven)	35 °C
Flow rate	1.5 ml/min
Wavelength	254 nm
Injection volume	20 µl (loop-type injector)
Detector sensitivity	set to obtain peak heights between 60% and 90% full-scale deflection
Retention time of deltamethrin	about 9 minutes

2.1.6 *Sample preparation and analysis*

Weigh (to the nearest 0.1 mg) two portions of the sample, prepared by grinding an entire tablet to contain about 15 mg of pure deltamethrin in each portion, into two 50-ml volumetric flasks and add 1 ml of distilled water to each flask. Dissolve in dioxane, make up to volume and mix thoroughly.

Pipette 10 ml of each suspension into two 50-ml volumetric flasks, make up to volume with iso-octane and mix thoroughly. Filter rapidly to prevent any solvent loss or centrifuge a part of this suspension. The extracts (S_1 and S_2), which must be clear, are used for the analysis. Keep the solutions in a thermostat bath at the same temperature as the calibration solution.

Inject 20-µl portions of calibration solution from one of the two flasks (C_1 or C_2) until the peak areas (or heights) of two successive injections agree to within 5%. Inject portions of the calibration solutions from flasks C_1 and C_2 and sample solutions from flasks S_1 and S_2 in succession in the following sequence: $C_1 S_1$, $C_2 S_1$, $C_1 S_2$, $C_2 S_2$.

2.1.7 *Calculation*

For each of the above four groups (i.e. C_1 versus S_1, C_2 versus S_1, C_1 versus S_2, and C_2 versus S_2) calculate the deltamethrin content.

Deltamethrin content (g/kg) = $\dfrac{a_2 \times m_1 \times P}{a_1 \times m_2}$

where a_1 = deltamethrin peak area (or height) of the calibration solution

a_2 = deltamethrin peak area (or height) of the sample solution

m_1 = mass of deltamethrin standard in the calibration solution (mg)

m_2 = one-fifth of the mass of the sample taken (mg)

P = purity of deltamethrin standard (g/kg)

The four results should agree to within 5% of their mean value. If not, repeat the analysis.

2.2 Deltamethrin R-isomer

2.2.1 Outline of method

Note: The method used to determine the deltamethrin *R*-isomer content differs slightly from the method described in the current WHO specification for deltamethrin technical and deltamethrin formulations (WP, EC, DP, UL, SC) in order to accommodate the extraction of deltamethrin active ingredient from the water-dispersible tablet.

The water-dispersible tablet sample is dissolved in a mixture of dioxane/water and iso-octane. The *R*-isomer content is determined by comparing the response of the sample with that of an *R*-isomer standard by high-performance liquid chromatography (HPLC), using a Nucleosil column (or equivalent) and a mixture of dioxane and iso-octane as the mobile phase.

2.2.2 Apparatus

Liquid chromatograph. The instrument should be one that is designed for use with stainless steel columns and is equipped with: a pumping system able to maintain a pressure of 15 MPa; a UV spectrophotometer detector able to measure UV absorbance at 254 nm; and a loop-type injector.

Liquid chromatographic column. The column should be a stainless steel tube 20 cm long and 4.0 mm in internal diameter, packed with Nucleosil 5 CN, 5 μm, Macherey Nagel (720007) or equivalent.

Recorder. 1-mV full-scale sensitivity, or integrator.

2.2.3 Reagents

Deltamethrin R-isomer standard. Analytical grade, of known purity.

1,4-Dioxane. HPLC grade. Check the peroxide content and purity if necessary. Dioxane is mixed with water at a concentration of 1.5 ml/l before use.

Iso-octane. HPLC grade.

Mobile phase. A degassed mixture of 6 ml of dioxane and 94 ml of iso-octane. Diluting solvent: dioxane–iso-octane 20:80 (v/v).

2.2.4 *Preparation of the calibration solution*
Weigh (to the nearest 0.1 mg) about 20 mg of deltamethrin *R*-isomer into a 50-ml volumetric flask. Dissolve and make up to volume with the mobile phase mixture. Pipette 10.0 ml of this solution into a 100-ml volumetric flask, make up to volume with the mobile phase mixture and mix thoroughly.

2.2.5 *Operating conditions for high-performance liquid chromatography*
The conditions given below are typical values and may have to be adapted to obtain optimal results from a given apparatus.

Column temperature	ambient
Flow rate	1.0–1.7 ml/min
Wavelength	254 nm
Injection volume	20 μl (loop-type injector)

Retention times:	
— *R*-isomer	about 8 minutes
— deltamethrin	about 9 minutes

2.2.6 *Sample preparation and analysis*
Weigh (to the nearest 0.1 mg) a sample prepared by grinding an entire tablet to contain about 200 mg of deltamethrin, into a glass-stoppered conical flask. Add 50 ml of diluting solvent. Extract for 15 minutes in an ultrasonic bath. Filter rapidly to avoid any solvent loss or alternatively centrifuge a part of the suspension. The extract, which must be clear, is used for the analysis.

Inject 20-μl portions of the calibration solution until the peak areas of two successive injections agree to within 5%. Inject the sample solution in duplicate. The results should agree to within 5%. If not, repeat the injections.

2.2.7 *Calculation*

$$R\text{-isomer content (g/kg)} = \frac{a_2 \times m_1 \times P}{a_1 \times m_2}$$

where a_1 = *R*-isomer peak area of the calibration solution
a_2 = *R*-isomer peak area of the sample solution
m_1 = mass of *R*-isomer standard in the calibration solution (mg)
m_2 = mass of the sample taken (mg)
P = purity of the *R*-isomer standard (g/kg)

The four results should agree to within 5% of their mean value. If not, repeat the analysis.

2.3 *Suspensibility*

2.3.1 *Outline of method*

A suspension of known concentration of deltamethrin in standard hard water is prepared by adding an entire water-dispersible tablet to standard hard water, poured into a 250-ml graduated cylinder, maintained at a constant temperature, and allowed to remain undisturbed for 30 minutes. The top nine-tenths are drawn off and the content of deltamethrin in the bottom one-tenth is determined, so allowing determination of the active ingredient mass still in suspension after 30 minutes.

2.3.2 *Apparatus*

A 250-ml graduated cylinder with a ground-glass stopper and a distance of 20.0–21.5 cm between the bottom and the 250-ml calibration mark.

A glass tube, about 40 cm long and about 5 mm in internal diameter, tapered at one end to an opening of 2–3 mm, the other end being connected to a suitable source of suction.

2.3.3 *Reagent*

WHO standard hard water (WHO method WHO/M/29; see Annex 2, section II).

2.3.4 *Procedure*

Weigh (to the nearest 0.1 mg) an entire water-dispersible tablet and place it in a 200-ml beaker. Add a volume of water at 30°C ± 2°C equal to at least twice the mass of the sample taken. Allow to stand for 30 seconds and then stir by hand for 30 seconds with a glass rod 4–6 mm in diameter, at not more than four revolutions per second, making no deliberate attempt to break up any lumps. Then immediately transfer the mixture quantitatively to the 250-ml graduated cylinder, using water at 30°C ± 2°C for rinsing, and again avoiding mechanical disintegration of lumps. Immediately add sufficient water at 30°C ± 2°C to bring the volume up to the 250-ml mark.

Insert the stopper and invert the cylinder end over end 30 times at the rate of one complete cycle every 2 seconds. This operation should be carried out as smoothly as possible, keeping the axis of rotation fixed. Allow the graduated cylinder to stand for 30 minutes in a water-bath at 30°C ± 2°C, taking care that the bath is free from vibrations. Should flocculation occur during the test, the material is unsatisfactory.

At the end of the 30-minute settling period, insert the glass tube into the cylinder and, with a minimum of disturbance, withdraw nine-tenths of the suspension (i.e. 225 ml) by means of the suction tube in a period of 10–15 seconds. This is achieved by maintaining the tip of the glass tube just below the sinking surface of the suspension. Discard the suspension withdrawn.

2.3.5 *Determination of deltamethrin in the retained one-tenth of the suspension*

2.3.5.1 *Apparatus*

See section 2.1.2 except that:

— the UV spectrophotometer detector must be able to measure UV absorbance at 230 nm,
— the column should be packed with a reverse phase (LiChrosorb RP18, 10 μm, or equivalent).

2.3.5.2 *Reagents*

See section 2.1.3 except that the mobile phase shall be a degassed mixture of 80 ml of acetonitrile and 20 ml of water (HPLC grade).

2.3.5.3 *Preparation of the calibration solution*

Weigh (to the nearest 0.1 mg) about 50 mg of deltamethrin standard into a 50-ml volumetric flask. Dissolve with acetonitrile (an ultrasonic bath can be used to accelerate dissolution). Dilute to volume with acetonitrile and mix thoroughly (if the volume of the sample is not 50 ml, correct the equation accordingly). Pipette 5 ml of the solution obtained into a 50-ml volumetric flask. Dilute to volume with a 50:50 (v/v) mixture of acetonitrile and water, and mix thoroughly.

2.3.5.4 *Operating conditions for high-performance liquid chromatography*

The conditions given below are typical values and may have to be adapted to obtain optimal results from a given apparatus.

Column temperature	ambient
Flow rate	1.0–1.5 ml/min
Wavelength	230 nm
Injection volume	20 μl (loop-type injector)
Retention time of deltamethrin	about 6 minutes

2.3.5.5 *Sample preparation and analysis*

Quantitatively transfer the retained one-tenth of the suspension to a 50-ml volumetric flask, rinsing several times with small quantities of acetonitrile. Dilute to about 1 cm below the mark and place the flask in an ultrasonic bath for 15 minutes to dissolve the deltamethrin (a volume contraction occurs) and wait for 15 minutes. Make up to volume with acetonitrile and mix thoroughly. Filter rapidly to avoid any solvent loss or centrifuge. The extract, which must be clear, is used for the analysis.

Inject 20 μl of the calibration solution until the peak areas (or heights) of two successive injections agree to within 5%. Inject the sample solution. The peak area (or height) for the sample solution must not differ by more than 20% from the peak area (or height) for the deltamethrin calibration solution. If it differs, adjust the volume of the sample to meet this requirement or prepare another calibration solution with an adapted deltamethrin content. If not, inject the calibration solution and the sample solution in duplicate.

2.3.6 *Calculation*

For each of the two calibration-solution-versus-sample-solution groups, calculate the deltamethrin content (m_1 mg) in the retained one-tenth of the suspension from the equation:

$$m_1 = \frac{a_1 \times m_0}{a_0 \times 10}$$

where a_0 = deltamethrin area (or height) of the calibration solution
$\quad\quad a_1$ = deltamethrin area (or height) of the sample solution
$\quad\quad m_0$ = mass of deltamethrin standard in the calibration solution (mg)

The values m_1 in the duplicate determinations must agree to within 5% of their mean. From the value obtained in section 2.1.7 for deltamethrin content, calculate the mass of deltamethrin in the initial sample taken for the suspensibility test.

$$\text{Suspensibility \%} = \frac{(m_2 - m_1) \times 111.1}{m_2}$$

where m_1 = mass of deltamethrin found in the retained one-tenth of the suspension (mg)
$\quad\quad m_2$ = mass of deltamethrin in the initial sample taken to prepare the suspension (mg)

2.4 *Heat stability treatment*

Test at 54 °C ± 2 °C for 14 days (CIPAC method MT 46.1) (*2*), unless other temperatures and times are requested.

After completion of the heat stability treatment, the samples should not be exposed to heat, bright sunlight or high atmospheric humidity.

If required, the test should be conducted in the commercial type pack.

Etofenprox emulsion, oil in water (EW)

Interim specification.

1. Specification

1.1 *Description*

The material shall consist of an emulsion of technical etofenprox in an aqueous phase together with any other necessary formulants. After gentle agitation the product shall be homogeneous and suitable for dilution in water. The technical etofenprox used in the manufacture of the emulsion, oil in water, shall comply with the requirements of specification WHO/IS/97.24.1 (*3*).

1.2 Chemical and physical requirements

The material, sampled from any part of the consignment (see method WHO/M/1 (*1*); see also Annex 1, section 3, of this report), shall comply with the requirements of section 1.1 and with the following requirements.

1.2.1 *Etofenprox content (g/kg basis)*

Nominal content	Tolerance permitted
Up to 25g/kg	±15% of the declared content
Above 25g/kg up to 100g/kg	±10% of the declared content
Above 100g/kg up to 250g/kg	±6% of the declared content

The average content of all the samples taken shall not be lower than the nominal content.

1.2.2 *pH*

The pH value of the concentrate, determined by CIPAC method MT 75 (*2*), shall lie in the range 6.0 to 8.0.

1.2.3 *Persistent foam*

The persistent foam at the top of 100ml of suspension prepared in WHO standard hard water (WHO method WHO/M/29; see Annex 2, section II) with 5ml of emulsion, oil in water, shall not exceed 10ml when tested by CIPAC method MT 47 (*2*).

1.2.4 *Flash-point*

The flash-point of the product determined by CIPAC method MT 12 (*2*) shall comply with all national and/or international transport regulations.

1.2.5 *Stability of the emulsion*

In standard soft water. Any separation, including creaming/oiling at the top and oiling/sedimentation at the bottom of 100 ml of emulsion prepared in WHO standard soft water (WHO method WHO/M/30; see Annex 2, section II) with 5 ml of emulsion, oil in water, shall not be visible when tested as described in WHO/M/13.R3 (*1*).

In standard hard water. Any separation, including creaming/oiling at the top and oiling/sedimentation at the bottom of 100 ml of emulsion prepared in WHO standard hard water (WHO method WHO/M/29; see Annex 2, section II) with 5 ml of emulsion, oil in water, shall not be visible when tested as described in WHO/M/13.R3 (*1*); see also Annex 1, section 3, of this report.

1.2.6 *Heat stability*

The emulsion, oil in water, after treatment as described in CIPAC method MT 46 (*2*), shall comply with the requirements of sections 1.2.2 and 1.2.5 of this specification.

1.3 **Packing and marking of packages**

Etofenprox emulsion, oil in water (EW), shall be packed in suitable clean containers, as specified in the order.

All packages shall bear, durably and legibly marked on the containers, the following:

— manufacturer's name
— "Etofenprox emulsion, oil in water"
— "Etofenprox.... g/kg"
— batch or reference number, and date of test
— net weight of contents
— date of manufacture
— instructions for dilution

and the following minimum cautionary notice:

Etofenprox is an insecticide with an action similar to pyrethroids, which act predominantly on the central nervous system. It may be hazardous if swallowed. Do not inhale spray mist. Avoid skin contact; wear protective gloves, clean protective clothing and a face mask (surgical type) when handling the product. Wash hands and exposed skin thoroughly after using.

Keep containers out of the reach of children and well away from foodstuffs and animal feed and their containers.

Etofenprox is toxic to aquatic wildlife. Avoid accidental contamination of water.

If poisoning occurs, call a physician. Treatment is symptomatic.

WHO has classified etofenprox as unlikely to present an acute hazard in normal use.

2. Methods of determining physical and chemical properties

2.1 *Etofenprox content*

2.1.1 *Outline of method*

The sample is dissolved in methanol/tetrahydrofuran (50:50, v/v) containing di-cyclohexyl phthalate as internal standard. Separation is carried out by gas–liquid chromatography with a flame ionization detector on a column of Chromosorb W-HP (or equivalent) coated with silicon AN-600. Etofenprox is determined by comparison with calibration solutions.

2.1.2 *Apparatus*

Gas–liquid chromatograph. Capable of operating over the range 100–300 °C with a flame ionization detector, injection port heater and on-column injection system, and equipped with a suitable recorder or electronic integrator.

Chromatographic column. Glass column 2 m long and 3 mm in internal diameter, packed with 55% silicone AN-600 on Chromosorb W-HP (60–80 mesh) or equivalent.

Injection volume. 1.0 μl.

Integrator. Automatic digital integrator or chromatography data system compatible with the gas chromatograph.

Before use, condition a freshly prepared column by purging with nitrogen overnight at 290 °C. During this operation the column must not be connected to the detector to avoid contamination by any initial "bleed" of the stationary phase.

2.1.3 *Reagents*

Methanol. Analytical grade.

Tetrahydrofuran. Analytical grade.

Internal standard. Di-cyclohexyl phthalate. Select for use a batch which, when chromatographed under the conditions given below for the determination of etofenprox, gives no peak with a similar retention time to etofenprox.

Etofenprox working standard. Pure analytical standard of known etofenprox content.

2.1.4 *Preparation of standard solutions*

Internal standard solution. Dissolve 1 g of di-cyclohexyl phthalate in 200 ml of methanol/tetrahydrofuran (50:50, v/v). It may be necessary to use an ultrasonic bath or to warm the mixture to assist dissolution. Before use, allow the solution to return to room temperature. Keep the solution in a thermostat bath if room temperature varies by more than 2 °C.

Etofenprox calibration solution. Weigh in duplicate (to the nearest 0.1 mg) about 0.06 g of etofenprox standard (M_A and M_B) into two 50-ml stoppered volumetric flasks. Add 10 ml of di-cyclohexyl phthalate internal standard solution, shake to dissolve the etofenprox and dilute to 50 ml with methanol/tetrahydrofuran (50:50, v/v) (solutions C_A and C_B). Keep the solutions in a thermostat bath if room temperature varies by more than 2 °C.

Prepare a solution with internal standard by dissolving about 0.06 g of standard in 50 ml of methanol/tetrahydrofuran (50:50, v/v) (solution C_O).

2.1.5 *Operating conditions*

The conditions given below are typical values and may have to be adapted to obtain optimal results from a given apparatus.

Temperatures

Column oven	230 °C
Injector	270 °C
Detector	270 °C

Adjust the column oven temperature, if required, to obtain retention time windows for etofenprox (approximately 19 minutes) and di-cyclohexyl phthalate (approximately 9.5 minutes), but do not exceed 300 °C.

Gas flow rates

Nitrogen	50 ml/min
Hydrogen	40 ml/min
Air	500 ml/min

2.1.6 *Sample preparation*

Sampling. Thoroughly mix the bulk material before taking at least 100 g as a subsample for analysis.

Preparation of the sample solutions. Thoroughly mix the material by the method given above for sampling.

Weigh in duplicate (to the nearest 0.1 mg) sufficient sample (_w_g) to contain about 0.06 g of etofenprox into two 50-ml stoppered volumetric flasks. Into each flask pipette 10 ml of di-cyclohexyl phthalate internal standard, shake the flasks thoroughly to dissolve the etofenprox and dilute to 50 ml with methanol/tetrahydrofuran (50:50, v/v) (solutions S_A and S_B).

Prepare a solution with internal standard by dissolving about 0.06 g of etofenprox in 50 ml of methanol/tetrahydrofuran (50:50, v/v) (solution S_O).

2.1.7 _Equilibration of the system_
Inject at least three portions of 1.0 µl of the etofenprox calibration solution C to equilibrate the system and use the data from these chromatograms to set the integrator parameters (if an integrator is being used) and also to assess the stability of the system.

Inject 1.0-µl portions of the internal standard solution and C_O and S_O solutions and check whether there are any interfering peaks from impurities. If there are, make any necessary corrections.

2.1.8 _Analysis of sample_
Carry out injections of 1.0 µl of the etofenprox calibration solutions C_A and C_B and sample solutions S_A and S_B and record either the integrated areas of the peaks or measure by triangulation (height × base). Injection sequence: C_{A1}, S_{A1}, S_{A2}, C_{B1}, C_{A2}, S_{B1}, S_{B2}, C_{B2}.

Calculate the relative response factors (f_1, f_2, etc.) for the pair of etofenprox calibration injections which bracket the sample injections, e.g. use C_{A1} and C_{B1} for sample injection S_{A1}, S_{A2}, etc., and obtain the mean response factor _f_.

$$\text{Relative response factor} = \frac{H_s}{I_r \times M \times P}$$

where H_s = area of etofenprox peak from the etofenprox calibration solution

I_r = area of di-cyclohexyl phthalate peak in the etofenprox calibration solution

M = mass of etofenprox analytical standard in the etofenprox calibration solution (g)

P = purity of the etofenprox analytical standard (g/kg)

The mass of internal standard is common to the etofenprox calibration solution and the sample solutions and has therefore been omitted.

Successive measurements of the response factors should agree to within 0.5% of their mean value. If not, repeat the analysis.

2.1.9 *Calculation*

Calculate the etofenprox content for each sample injection, e.g. S_{A1}, using the following equation:

$$\text{Etofenprox content (g/kg)} = \frac{I\,I_w}{f \times I_q \times \underline{w}}$$

where f = mean relative response factor
H_w = area of etofenprox peak in the sample solution
I_q = area of the di-cyclohexyl phthalate peak in the sample solution
$\underline{w}$ = mass of sample (g)

Take the mean of the four values corresponding to the four injections S_{A1}, S_{A2}, S_{B1}, S_{B2}. Calculate the etofenprox content of the sample as the mean of the four determinations as follows:

Sample injection	*Use relative response factor from*	*Etofenprox*	
S_{A1}	C_{A1} and C_{B1}	$Q\%$	$\Big\}\ U\%$
S_{A2}	C_{A1} and C_{B1}	$R\%$	
S_{B1}	C_{A2} and C_{B2}	$S\%$	$\Big\}\ V\%$
S_{B2}	C_{A2} and C_{B2}	$T\%$	

Q and R, and S and T should agree to within 0.5% of their mean values (U and V). U and V should agree to within 1% of their mean values. Take the mean of the two values U and V as the total etofenprox content.

II. New test methods

Method for the determination of tablet integrity (WHO/M/27)

1. Outline of method

The integrity of the tablet formulation is assessed by rotating a pre-determined number of tablets in a tablet friability tester.

2. Apparatus

Balance

Tablet friability tester. Equipped with a specific rotating disc.

3. Procedure

Weigh the tablets (see Note 1 below). Introduce the tablets into the rotating disc. Replace the cover, then fix the rotating disc to the tester.

Set the rotation speed and the duration of the test. Start the rotation. At the end of the rotation, report any broken tablets; collect and weigh the tablets (see Note 2 below).

4. **Calculation**

Tablet integrity is determined by calculating the degree of attrition according to the formula

$$\text{Degree of attrition (\%)} = \frac{(M_1 - M_2)}{M_1} \times 100$$

where M_1 = weight of the tablets before rotation
M_2 = weight of the tablets after rotation

Report the degree of attrition to the nearest 0.1% and specify the following conditions:

— specification of rotating disc
— rotation speed
— duration of test.

Note 1. Weigh 10 tablets if the weight of a single tablet is 5 g. Weigh two tablets if the weight of a single tablet is >5 g.

Note 2. The test is declared failed if broken tablets are collected after completion of the rotation.

Method for the determination of tablet disintegration time (WHO/M/28)

1. **Outline of method**

One entire water-dispersible tablet is added to a defined volume of water and mixed by stirring to form a suspension. After standing for a determined period of time the suspension is passed through a 2000-µm sieve. The ease with which the water-dispersible tablet is disintegrated in water is determined by the absence of residue left on the sieve.

2. **Apparatus**

Beaker. 1000 ml, with a diameter of 102 ± 2 mm (low form).

Stirrer motor. With speed control.

Stainless steel stirrer. Propeller type, with four fixed stirrer blades set at an angle of 45°. Particular attention should be given to the construction of the stirrer; its dimensions should conform to those shown in Fig. 1.

Sieve. 200-mm diameter test sieve with 2000-µm aperture size.

Figure 1
A propeller-type stirrer

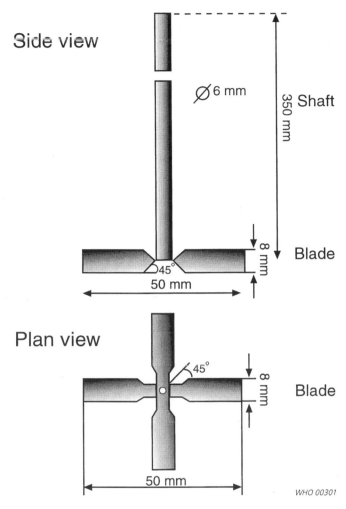

Side view

Ø6 mm

350 mm Shaft

8 mm Blade

45°

50 mm

Plan view

45°

8 mm Blade

50 mm

WHO 00301

3. **Reagent**

WHO standard hard water (WHO method WHO/M/29; see page 68).

4. **Procedure**

Fill the beaker with 1000 ml of standard hard water at 30 °C ± 2 °C. The stirrer should be centrally located in the beaker and positioned in such a way that the lower edges of the stirrer blades are 60 mm above the base of the beaker. The pitch of the stirrer blades and the direction of rotation are such that the propeller pushes the water upwards. Add the tablet to the water without stirring. Wait for 1 minute. Switch on the stirrer with the speed set to about 300 rev/min and continue the stirring for 2.5 minutes. Then switch off the stirrer and immediately pour the suspension through the 2000-μm sieve. Rinse the beaker out with 50 ml of standard hard water and pour the residue through the 2000-μm sieve.

5. **Test result**

The absence of residue retained on the 2000-μm sieve indicates that the disintegration of the water-dispersible tablet is complete.

Preparation of WHO standard hard water (WHO/M/29)

Dissolve 0.304 g of anhydrous calcium chloride and 0.139 g of magnesium chloride hexahydrate in distilled water and make up to 1 litre. This provides water with a hardness of 342 mg/l, calculated as calcium carbonate.

Preparation of WHO standard soft water (WHO/M/30)

Dilute one part of WHO standard hard water prepared as described in WHO method WHO/M/29, the hardness of which is 342 mg/l, with nine parts of distilled water to give a hardness of 34.2 mg/l.

References

1. *Specifications for pesticides used in public health: insecticides, molluscicides, repellents, methods*, 7th ed. Geneva, World Health Organization, 1997 (unpublished document WHO/CTD/WHOPES/97.1; available on request from Communicable Disease Control, Prevention and Eradication, World Health Organization, 1211 Geneva 27, Switzerland).

2. Dobrat W, Martijn A. *Physico-chemical methods for technical and formulated pesticides, CIPAC Handbook, Vol. F.* Cambridge, Black Bear Press, 1995.

3. *Interim specifications for pesticides used in public health.* Geneva, World Health Organization, 1997 (unpublished document WHO/CTD/WHOPES/97.7; available on request from Communicable Disease Control, Prevention and Eradication, World Health Organization, 1211 Geneva 27, Switzerland).